Testimonials About the Author

"**Dr. Hirani is giving me my life back**. Maybe that sounds a bit dramatic, but it is true. I've been living with a chronic illness for over twenty years now. My pain continues to diminish, and my chronic fatigue condition, which I had gone to see Dr. Hirani for, has also improved tremendously. She has done specific functional medical tests and has corrected nutritional deficiencies and hormonal imbalances in me as well, which has also contributed to my successful path toward healing."

"I first met Dr. Hirani two years ago and discovered soon after that **she exemplifies what a physician ought to be**."

"I am so grateful to have met Dr. Karima Hirani for many reasons. She is a wonderful human being, committed to a person's well-being by using the least invasive procedures. **My quality of life is a hundred times better** since she started helping me."

"Dr. Hirani truly is, as the **Yelp star rating** says, "**As good as it gets!**" Dr. Hirani found the underlying cause of my life-threatening illness that several other doctors fumbled the ball with when trying to diagnose me. My Lyme disease had gone unchallenged at that time for about seven and a half years. God has used my illness to humble me and cause me to appreciate Him, life, and people more. God also brought Dr. Hirani into my life and I am the better for it."

"Dr. Hirani is also a **social activist** and does great work with feeding the homeless and people in need as the lead organizer at ICSC Food Pantry, where she maintains that same level of care. She volunteers her time to educate on various health topics such as nutrition, diabetes, and heart disease to the underserved communities throughout Los Angeles."

"In ninth grade, I broke my upper arm during a wrestling practice. It was a clean break through the ball at the head of humerus. I was told this was a life-altering injury that would only get more chronically painful as time passed, and eventually require a total shoulder replacement. Despite the injury, I excelled in football up to the NFL level. It was a proud accomplishment but expedited both the degeneration and pain in the joint, leaving me in a constant pain of four-to-seven (ten being unbearable). I tried several different therapies to reduce the pain and got intermittent relief at best, but never long-lasting results.

I met Dr. Hirani in a mutual Mastermind group where she introduced me to Ozone Therapy Treatment. After just a SINGLE treatment my pain levels have been consistently between a one and two over a year later. It has truly been incredible. **Ever since she treated me, I have recommended Dr Hirani to all of my [athlete] friends who are suffering from pain— Dr. Hirani's oxygen-ozone therapy treatment works!**"

"Dr. Hirani has been a **miracle worker** replacing fear and despair with tears of joy and peace with our boys. We are eternally grateful to this doctor, woman, and mother."

"I had been suffering from an ongoing back issue with severe injuries to my spine due to a car accident years ago. Dr. Hirani and her medical staff gave me a **world-class level of care**. I would call her **'Wonder Woman,'** but for me she was a **major Blessing**. Thank you, Dr. Karima Hirani, I don't know how my back would feel and skin would look without you."

"I saw Dr. Hirani several years ago and she tested me for a number of items. The results showed I had heavy metals in my system and chelation was started. I also began LDA [low-dose allergen] treatment and have continued to do so over the years. Among other problems, I was suffering from tinnitus, and the PEMF treatment she offers is the only thing that provided relief. **My health has never been better** in my life both professionally and personally. I have Dr. Hirani to thank, and I tell her this every time I visit. **She is the best physician I have ever met**. I got my life back after years and years of illness, and the LDA shots have kept me healthy."

"Just amazing! Very thorough medical exams from blood test and allergy testing to nutrition coaching, Dr. Hirani has been a **Godsend to our family**. She helped my husband who has been in pain for years with an autoimmune disease. He has now been pain free for two years—it's amazing and such a blessing. Thank you, Dr. Hirani, [Nurse] Toby, and all the staff! You are all just **what medical professionals should be**."

WHAT YOUR DOCTOR DIDN'T TELL YOU

HOW COMPLEMENTARY AND ALTERNATIVE MEDICINE CAN HELP YOUR PAIN

Karima Hirani, MD, MPH

Master of Public Health in Nutrition
Board Certification in Family Medicine
Board Certification in Clinical Homeopathy

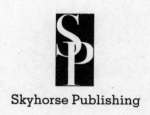

Skyhorse Publishing

Skyhorse Publishing books may be purchased in bulk at special discounts for sales promotion, corporate gifts, fund-raising, or educational purposes. Special editions can also be created to specifications. For details, contact the Special Sales Department, Skyhorse Publishing, 307 West 36th Street, 11th Floor, New York, NY 10018 or info@skyhorsepublishing.com.

Skyhorse® and Skyhorse Publishing® are registered trademarks of Skyhorse Publishing, Inc.®, a Delaware corporation.

Visit our website at www.skyhorsepublishing.com.

10 9 8 7 6 5 4 3 2 1

Library of Congress Cataloging-in-Publication Data is available on file.

Cover design by Kai Texel

Print ISBN: 978-1-5107-7071-3
Ebook ISBN: 978-1-5107-7072-0

Printed in the United States of America

This book is dedicated to all my pain patients, who have been my greatest teachers, and for the 1.5 billion chronic pain sufferers globally.

Table of Contents

Disclaimer

The advice and recommendations in this book are not meant to replace those of your own doctor or health provider. Please seek your doctor's advice before embarking on any treatments discussed in this book.

All efforts to confirm the accuracy of the information contained in this book have been made as of its publication date. Health information and opinions change, so the reader should be made aware that reading information contained in this book at any date after its original publication may be outdated or incorrect. The author and publisher disclaim any liability of health outcomes that may result from trying any of the interventions discussed in this book.

All statements made in this book about products, drugs, nutraceuticals, and treatments have not been evaluated by the US Food and Drug Administration (FDA).

All names of patients have been changed to protect their privacy. All testimonials in this book are based on the experience of these few people, and you may not have the same experience. In accordance with the Federal Trade Commission (FTC) guidelines concerning the use of endorsements and testimonials in advertising, the testimonials in this book reflect the personal experiences and opinions of these individuals, and again, they may not represent what every consumer may personally experience.

No part of this book may be reproduced or utilized in any form or by any means, electronic or mechanical, including recording, duplicating, or by informational storage or retrieval system without the author's prior written consent.

Please note: Neural trigger point therapy, oxygen-ozone therapy, and mesenchymal stem cell therapy are not FDA approved and not covered by insurance. Pulsed electromagnetic field (PEMF) therapy and platelet-rich plasma (PRP) therapy are approved for use (in some cases), but also are not covered by insurance. The use of stem cells or stem cell–rich tissues, as well as mobilization of stem cells by any means (e.g., pharmaceutical, mechanical, or herbal based), is not FDA approved to treat, cure, or make any medical condition mentioned in this book better.

The Big Picture

- If you have recurrent aches and pains, then you are one of **fifty million American adults** who **suffer from chronic pain**. You also probably know that the outcomes of pain management are dismal.
- **Anxiety, depression, insomnia, and stress** are four of the most common symptoms that accompany chronic pain—and they **are treatable!**
- In 2019, Big Pharma spent **$3.7 billion** on television advertising in the United States.
- **Three of the most frequently advertised medicines are for pain or arthritis**: Humira®, Lyrica®, and Xeljanz®. Yet none of these drugs promise total relief.

So, why are we being told that we need to learn to live with pain?

The Prognosis:

- **Diet can bring about a 25–30 percent improvement** of your pain when combined with exercise.
- Not all knee pain is due to osteoarthritis, so **you may not need that knee replacement!**
- **Mother Nature's PEMFs** (pulsed electromagnetic fields) work to **resolve pain**.
- A **secret treatment** led former **President Kennedy's** White House staff physician, Dr. Janet Travell, to be known as the "Trigger Queen" of trigger point injection therapy.
- **Oxygen-ozone therapy succeeds in pain management** when other treatments fail.

- You can manage your gut-brain axis to **control and influence inflammation and pain!**
- Learn how the **allergy elimination diet** used by Dr. Hirani can help reduce your pain!

After achieving successful outcomes for thousands of pain sufferers, Dr. Hirani states this with confidence:

"You don't need to let another day go by with pain."

Foreword

by Dr. Gregorio Martínez-Sánchez

The International Association for the Study of Pain defines pain as "an unpleasant sensory and emotional experience associated with actual or potential tissue damage or described in terms of such damage." More than 20 percent of adults worldwide experience different types of chronic pain, which are frequently associated with several comorbidities and a decrease in quality of life. Several approved painkillers are available, but current analgesics are often hampered by insufficient efficacy and/or severe adverse effects. Although advances have been made in treatments for chronic pain, it remains inadequately controlled for many people. Adverse effects and complications of analgesic drugs, such as addiction, kidney failure, and gastrointestinal bleeding also limit their use. Consequently, novel strategies for safe, highly efficacious treatments are very desirable, particularly for chronic pain.

The experience of pain is characterized by tremendous interindividual variability. Multiple biological and psychosocial variables contribute to these individual differences in pain, including demographic variables, genetic factors, and psychosocial processes. Understanding these mosaics is critically important in order to provide optimal pain treatment, and future research to further elucidate the nature of these biopsychosocial interactions is needed in order to provide more informed and personalized pain care. In this sense, this book opens up a range of possibilities and alternatives to pain treatment.

Complementary and integrative medicine (CIM), also known as complementary and alternative medicine (CAM) in the United States, encompasses both Western-style medicine and complementary health approaches as a new combined approach to treat a variety of clinical conditions. Chronic pain is the leading indication for use of CIM, and about 33 percent of adults and 12 percent of children in the United States have used it in this context. CIM offers a multimodality treatment approach that can tackle the multidimensional nature of pain with fewer or no serious adverse effects. In addition, novel methods to control pain, such as the use of growth factors derived from platelets and stem cells, can be integrated into the treatment of this disorder.

This book reviews the main forms of chronic pain: postoperative (surgical) pain, pelvic pain, neuropathic pain, joint pain, chronic low back pain, and headaches and focuses on the use of CIM and innovative therapeutic managements, such as dietary interventions, pulsed electromagnetic field therapy, stimulating neural trigger point therapy, oxygen-ozone therapy, platelet-rich plasma, and stem cells. Dr. Hirani, with an integrative approach, makes a great contribution to this field and in the search for a better quality of life for patients.

> "Of pain you could wish only one thing: that it should stop.
> Nothing in the world was so bad as physical pain. In the face of
> pain there are no heroes."
>
> George Orwell, *1984*

Gregorio Martínez-Sánchez, PharmD, PhD
President of the ISCO3
(International Scientific Committee of Ozone Therapy)

Foreword

by Dr. Tracy Brobyn

It takes a lot of effort to become a doctor. That effort includes years of grueling training, sleepless nights, boatloads of money, and self-sacrifice. It stands to reason that if you are willing to get through it, the rainbow at the end of that long, dark tunnel ought to be pretty amazing. Now imagine that there is no rainbow—or worse—the tunnel ends in a sort of bleak and drizzled fog. This fog is what many of us encounter upon entering traditional medicine. You only have to get six months into medical school before you realize that the vast majority of our tools are mostly drugs and/or surgery. Between years two and three, you realize that most drugs really only mask symptoms (if they work at all). By residency, you come to the dismal realization that most of your patients are going to be stuck taking these drugs for the rest of their lives, whether that's three years or thirty. At the end of the day, physicians go into medicine to heal and, dare I say it, CURE. Our current state of affairs in medicine is anything but that. However, there is a glimmer of light in the midst of that fog, and with this book, Dr. Hirani cuts through it, revealing both the rainbow and the pot of gold. If you are a patient in pain, that pot of gold can be yours.

In fact, for most people, it is not only possible to be pain free, but it also takes far less time to get there than you would think. In my twenty-five years of treating patients, it has only been since embracing the concept of healing energy interferences that I have been able to achieve what most of my patients refer to as "the magic." These techniques are straightforward and can include something as simple as small procaine injections into scars, injections over areas of energy dysregulation, or injecting healing substances like ozone into damaged tissue. The really amazing thing about it, though, is that it isn't magic. It's deeply rooted in scientific principles that have been well established in the medical community for decades (if not centuries).

While researching my first paper on neural therapy ("Neural Therapy: An Overlooked Game Changer for Patients Suffering Chronic Pain?" published in the *Journal of Pain & Relief*), I was astounded to discover that these principles began with Nobel Prize–winning scientists such as Neher and Sakmann. These gentlemen discovered that there is fluid between the cells in the body that contains electrically active compounds called ions. These ions allow ALL CELLS in the body to be in contact with each other (not unlike an elaborate Wi-Fi network). This work was further developed by another Nobel Prize winner named Pischinger, who proved that a complex system of compounds exists within the intercellular matrix, which fills the space between cells. This complex system of connectivity is responsible for regulation throughout the whole body. Changes in the body due to an interference in the system, such as a scar, inflamed muscle trigger point, or injured nerve will lead to disruption throughout the system. Local anesthetics and ozone can treat these disruptions by resetting those ions and compounds, which is not unlike rebooting your computer.

I like to embrace the concept of an onion when I think of healing patients. Pain and most other chronic conditions are a result of several different problems (a so-called multifactorial root cause). This thinking over the years is what has led me to many of the same conclusions as Dr. Hirani. There need to be several weapons in your medical arsenal that go above and beyond surgery and drugs. These weapons need to address disruption of energy, disruption of muscle, and deficiency of oxygen. Dr. Hirani does an exceptional job in this book of not only providing a wonderful explanation for why these treatments work (pulsed electromagnetic field therapy, neural trigger point therapy, and oxygen-ozone therapy), but also how they are practically used in the healing of patients at the point of care. Each layer of that "onion" needs to be addressed whether it is a belly button piercing, progesterone deficiency during the second half of the menstrual cycle, or wheat intolerance, all of which together can lead to abdominal pain and bloating. All layers of the onion must be addressed in order to get the patient to the cure. Dr. Hirani understands the dedication and drive that is required to achieve this level of success, and I could not be more pleased to have her invaluable insights available to the public.

Pain is a devastating blight on our current society. It permeates all aspects of illness and leads to depression, disability, and hopelessness. As most Americans are aware, especially in light of our current opioid crisis, drugs are not the answer. In fact, they are killing us. We need alternatives NOW—alternatives that work. That takes a doctor who not only thinks outside the box, but outside the building! As I said before, it takes a lot of effort to become a doctor. However, it takes a wealth of imagination and courage to become a doctor who gets to heal. Dr. Hirani shows us in this book that a resolution is not only possible but expected. And that can only mean one thing—that rainbow was there the whole time.

Tracy L. Brobyn, MD, FAAFP, DABMA
The Chung Institute of Integrative Medicine
The Won Sook Chung Foundation
Assistant Clinical Professor, Department of Family Medicine
Rowan University School of Osteopathic Medicine

Preface

I have been practicing complementary and alternative medicine (CAM) and integrative medicine for over two decades. As a board-certified family physician with a Master of Public Health degree in nutrition, I am formally trained in complementary and alternative pain solutions. I apply the techniques I have learned to successfully treat thousands of chronic pain patients just like you who benefit from long-term results. The bottom line is that *you shouldn't be suffering from your pain*. If you have suffered from chronic pain, then you know how it can rob you of many things that life has to offer. I deeply believe that all my patients, and you, dear reader, deserve to know about the scientifically vetted techniques that can help manage and get rid of your pain.

My intention in writing this book is to present these approaches to pain management, which, while they may be new to the reader, have actually been around for decades. My hope is that you will benefit from my experience with an enhanced understanding of your own pain and that it will enable you to make an informed and better choice about the modalities that would work best for you.

This book also offers a counterpoint to some of the misrepresentations the medical establishment tells patients about their chronic pain. A reputable medical journal, *Clinical Case Reports*, sums up the current status of pain sufferers: "As there is no cure or medical intervention that can fully resolve their problems, individuals with chronic pain must often deal with a future having an unforeseen course."[1]

In other words, the above-referenced article is explaining to doctors that they must set realistic expectations about their patient's pain. The implication is that the pain is not going to go away completely, and the patient will just have to learn to live with it. The article goes on to say, "There is a growing awareness that the successful treatment of chronic pain must be multifaceted and individualized, as psychosocial factors can affect the total life situation of the sufferer."[2]

Indeed, if you suffer from chronic pain, you know how much it affects so many—if not all—aspects of your life. *I want to underscore that there are many well-intentioned doctors out there who meet this need for treatment by offering a combination of therapies.* These often include pain medications augmented with other methods, such as tai chi, cognitive-behavioral therapy, or psychotherapy. Quite often, they are successful in providing their patients with the means to cope and maintain some semblance of a normal life.

On the opposite end of the spectrum, there are doctors who have nothing to offer but pain medications. However, what I see in my office almost daily is how specific pain treatments can bring about true and lasting resolution of pain. The treatments I use are scientific, safe, and can provide instantaneous results for some patients. If there is one thing you get out of this book, I want you to understand that no matter what kind of pain you suffer —from headaches or sciatica to fibromyalgia or neuropathic pain—*it is all treatable.* You will be relieved to hear that *it's possible to get your life back!*

By now, I'm sure you're asking, "If my chronic pain is treatable, then why hasn't my doctor told me about these complementary and alternative medical treatments?" The answer is complicated. First, the medical establishment mandates that all treatments can only become widely accepted once they have undergone successful and rigorous, double-blind, placebo-controlled studies. The challenge facing those of us in integrative medicine and alternative healthcare is that performing these types of research studies requires an investment of millions of dollars. The biggest obstacle is that only the Big Pharmaceutical industry has deep enough pockets to fund these kinds of studies on chronic pain.

Since there are little or no major potential profits in studying non-patentable or non-pharmacological treatments, the required studies that would deliver game-changing treatments never get funded, and thus, never become mainstream treatment modalities. As a result, perfectly effective therapies that have already undergone extensive scientific scrutiny—here in the United States and in other countries—will never become common knowledge or available to your doctor or you. In truth, your doctor doesn't even know about these treatments herself. So how could she tell you about them? She doesn't know that relief from chronic or acute pain is achievable with minimal training on her part and at a very low cost to the patient in comparison to a lifetime of paying for pain medications and suffering.

As I write this, we are at a crossroads in the treatment of chronic pain. I was motivated to write this book to provide an overview of pioneering approaches that have been available for years—and some even for decades—but which are not usually written about for the general public. Other books about pain management describe coping strategies for those with chronic pain or are written in the form of self-help books that promise to help you accept your lot in life as a chronic pain sufferer.

My approach to pain management, which I call The Golden Triad for Pain Relief™, features three overlooked therapies that are foundational to our successful treatments at the Hirani Integrative Medical Center: pulsed electromagnetic field (PEMF) therapy, neural trigger point therapy, and oxygen-ozone therapy.

This book is for chronic pain sufferers who have lost all hope as well as those who are the opposite and refuse to accept that pain is a life sentence. So, if you haven't had any success with traditional pain treatments, or you've had too many side effects from pain medications and treatments, then this book is for you. If you are curious to learn about some pain treatment strategies not previously known to you, or you don't fully trust what your doctor is telling you, then this book is also for you.

Finally, if you are a doctor or healthcare practitioner who wants to help patients and knows that there must be something better than what is currently offered for pain management, then this book is certainly for you, too!

Karima Hirani, MD, MPH
Culver City, California

Acknowledgments

First and foremost, I thank God for guiding me on the path to becoming a physician, and a holistic one at that.

Second, I want to thank all my patients, who are my most excellent teachers and inspiration! When I cannot help your pain, I see it as a failure, and it motivates me to continue to innovate and search for solutions that are natural and will help you with the least amount of side effects.

I am also grateful to my many teachers in the various fields of pulsed electromagnetic field therapy, neural trigger point therapy, and oxygen-ozone therapy, including, but not limited to, Dr. Dennis Harper, Dr. Dietrich Klinghardt, Dr. Adriana Schwartz, Dr. Robert Rowen, Dr. Glenn Sperbeck, Dr. Frank Shallenberger, and Dr. Gregorio Martínez-Sánchez.

My appreciation is extended to Kevin Stein for helping me with editing, marketing, and more. I want to thank Teri Arranga for her tireless editing efforts toward making the information presented as accurate as possible. I wish to thank an anonymous person who has also played a significant role from the beginning to the end of making this book possible.

I also want to express my ongoing gratitude to my mom and dad, who grew up with no education or money, came to this country as immigrants, and worked hard so that I could become a doctor and accomplish what they couldn't have ever imagined for themselves. They are forever my greatest role models for hard work, sharing, and selflessness.

How to Use This Book

Many readers will naturally want to skip ahead to chapters related to their particular chronic pain condition. That's a fine way to approach the book. But if you choose to do so, please make sure you **read the first three chapters** because they lay the foundation for understanding the historical and current background on the subject of pain management.

In particular, the first several chapters address why today's medical establishment and Big Pharmaceutical companies can sometimes present challenges to advances in treating pain. Chapter 3 addresses the fundamentals of why proper nutrition is a key to alleviating pain—*even if that's all that you do!*

For readers who are interested in more information about my sources and additional scientific references, I've included these in the appendices.

Finally, if you are afraid of needles—even the small acupuncture-like ones—you may still benefit from the chapters concerning eliminating pain through diet and pulsed electromagnetic field therapy, so I encourage you to skip ahead to those sections.

Most of all, your feedback about how useful you've found this book is extremely meaningful to me, and your suggestions will be helpful for future editions. So, please feel free to email me at inquiry@drhirani.com, and thank you for being one of my respected readers!

CHAPTER 1

There is No Money in
Curing Your Pain

"Money often costs too much."
—Ralph Waldo Emerson

You can find relief from your pain, but pursuing traditional routes probably won't get you there. Why? The reason is simple: *There's no money in it.* The unfortunate truth is that the profiteering of others is what controls how you can deal with your pain. I recently attended a pain management conference and was horrified when I heard experts saying things like, "Even with the right combination of pain medications, your patients can only expect 50 percent improvement in their pain."

Think about it. You are in a pithole of pain; you seek out medical help, but when you go to your doctor, she tells you that the likelihood of success over your pain is only 50 percent. You trust her, so you buy into that. The establishment has told you not to expect much. So, you have no reason not to believe in this message, especially when it's conveyed by medical professionals. You might end up saying with resignation, "Well, that's as good as I'm ever going to get."

You can't blame these experts entirely for what they think are realistic expectations about pain management. You've been told, "Pain medications may help a little, but there are no guarantees." And all of us have accepted this. As a society, we've come to believe what our doctors tell us and settle for less than what we deserve.

This has not been my professional experience. What I've seen is that many patients at Hirani Integrative Medicine Center have received relief from their pain.

As a result, I have pursued research over the years to answer the following questions:

- Why do we come to blindly accept what we are told *without questioning* these highly esteemed institutions?
- Why are we told that we have to learn to live with painful conditions from which *we can never fully recover*?"

Just like in any good murder mystery, you should always follow the money.

A Profit-Driven System

The enemy we all face is a profit-driven system. Name any major problem that exists in our society today, and it almost always has to do with money. Follow the money, and you will usually find the answer to the root cause of these problems. The tragic fact is that there is little profit in getting you back to a pain-free life. It may sound cynical, but many companies profit by you continuing to experience enough pain that keeps you going back to the doctor. What eventually happens is a vicious cycle of pain, pain management, buying more drugs, and becoming reliant on a system and drug industry that doesn't seem to really want you to get better. It's that simple—if you got better, then you probably wouldn't need them anymore.

More than fifty million American adults suffer from chronic pain.[3] The traditional outcomes of pain management are utterly dismal. It's not just my opinion—this statement is based on statistics, and any expert in pain management will agree. The cost of chronic pain is nearly $600 billion in the United States annually, a sum which includes overall treatment costs as well as loss of productivity.[4] The latter means loss of income resulting from employees who are unable to perform work due to their pain.

I know that statistics aren't helpful when all you know and care about is that you hurt and are angry that you hurt so much. I've had patients who've tried everything for their pain, spent thousands of dollars themselves (or, hopefully, through insurance), made countless doctor's office visits, often suffered years of pain, and are no better than when the pain began. I agree that you should be angry.

But you need to ask yourself a logical question: "If this vicious cycle is so ineffective, why does the status quo of pain management remain unquestioned?" The reality is that it exists due to your continued reliance and blind faith. More importantly, it remains unchallenged based on your willingness to continue to pay for less-than-satisfactory results.

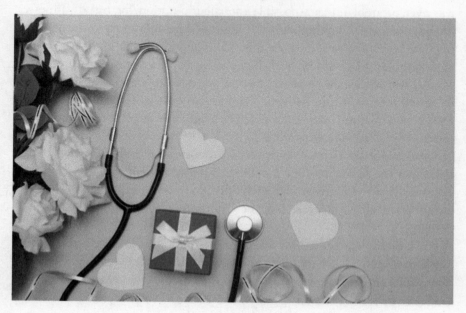

The First Bribe in Medical School

When I think about my journey to integrative medicine, it really started during my first year of medical school. At the time, as an aspiring physician, I'd already completely bought into the system. Little did I know, I was experiencing a watershed moment in my career that would only make sense some years later.

We were listening to the professor speak on microbiology in a large lecture hall. Suddenly, she was interrupted by the appearance of a messenger who began informing us about the "free" stethoscopes from Eli Lilly (a large pharmaceutical company) that would be made available to all of us following class. As a young student, I didn't think much of it at first. We were still staring at the messenger as the professor began writing in huge letters on the chalkboard: YOUR FIRST BRIBE. At the time, I didn't understand what she meant by that provocative statement, but it somehow stuck in my mind.

As I was making my transition eight years later to becoming an integrative medicine doctor, it finally hit me. My medical education was a "bribe" of sorts: learn pathology, microbiology, pathophysiology, and then pharmacology (how drugs work); learn about the disease, then know when to prescribe a certain drug—and nothing more. No diet, herb, or supplement was ever brought up as a possible therapeutic option for certain illnesses. Throughout my schooling and training, we were constantly rewarded with free lunches in the hospitals. As practicing physicians, we graduated to free drug samples, free dinners, and shows at fancy restaurants or theaters.

All the while, we thought that we were being trained to do the best we could for our future patients. "You are an excellent doctor!" I was told. However, I realized over time that the medicines mostly treat the symptoms—*they don't cure the disease.*

You might say that the entire medical profession has been persuaded to believe in the status quo, me included. But guess what? So have you! After all these years of modern medicine and pharmaceuticals, we still have no cure for prevailing illnesses like the common cold and allergies as well as diabetes.

For example, the best we have for allergies are Benadryl® and similar antihistamines, which treat the allergy symptoms, but nothing more. We doctors are in the business of prescribing medicines for symptomatic relief. *Unfortunately, there's absolutely no money in curing chronic pain.*

Patients are also bribed. They are told to lower their expectations—that their pain is not going to get a whole lot better—so no one is ultimately held accountable. And all you do is keep going back to the doctor. At the end of the day, the only way to be satisfied is to have such low expectations that you're never disappointed by the largely ineffective treatment you receive.

CHAPTER 2

You Are Bribed about Your Pain

"Paying good coin to bad men."
—George R. R. Martin, *Fire & Blood*

We're taught to trust doctors without question. Somehow, the initials "MD" that traditionally follow doctors' names makes them seem infallible—if not superheroes. Doctors put on that white coat, and they are suddenly regarded as great founts of wisdom with profound knowledge of everything medical. Doctors are anointed by our society as supreme professionals, and everyone is supposed to hang onto our every word in total belief and trust.

When it comes to treating pain, doctors largely know what is dished out to them by the Establishment—that is, unless they have pursued continuing education in alternative and integrative modalities. Like the medical students and doctors in the previous chapter, you've also been bribed when you have low expectations for full recovery from your pain. But you're not to blame. You are just responding to what you've been told by professionals who are put on a pedestal by our society. At a certain point, you will be fed up with hurting without recourse and be moved to seek help based on fresh information that promises hope.

Your doctor didn't tell you about alternative solutions that are available to you when they said that you may have to live with your pain. Ideally, this pronouncement would have been followed by a combination of prescribed strategies that delivered the "best" results you could have. Chances are that your doctor most likely had nothing much to offer for your pain. When left untreated, pain can have enormous consequences for virtually every aspect of your life—from family and work to play. Anxiety, depression, insomnia, and stress are four of the most common symptoms that accompany chronic pain.

The stress is not surprising, given our inability to function normally or to work when we are in pain. When you are unable to work, earning money can be very difficult. Without income, the ability to pay for life's necessities can become a real challenge and even affect our very survival.

When stress levels go up, our closest relationships are also impacted. In fact, the likelihood of divorce among patients suffering from chronic pain is higher than for people without it. Plus, every day that you experience pain is another day you have lost to poor quality of life and unhappiness. I am convinced from my successful practice that it doesn't have to be this way. Let's begin by taking a look at the most common forms that pain takes.

Headaches

The typical headache is something that all of us have experienced at one time or another. How many of you have a headache just by reading these first chapters—especially about how the establishment profits from your pain? So, how do you treat such a headache? Well, the first thing pain sufferers usually do is to take a pill. We've all been trained—or, as I like to say, "bribed"—to rely on a pill for most common ailments. For example, I bet if you go and open up your medicine cabinet right now, you will find several different types of Excedrin® or other similar medications for different types of headaches.

You probably didn't know that Excedrin® Extra Strength has the same ingredients as Excedrin® Migraine. Then, there is the Excedrin® PM Headache, which has Benadryl® instead of the caffeine that is in the Excedrin® Extra Strength version. Excedrin® Tension Headache and Excedrin® Sinus Headache (currently unavailable) make up the different headache sub-brands of Excedrin®. And let's not forget Excedrin® Back and Body, which has the same ingredients as did Excedrin® Menstrual Complete (which is no longer available). So, folks, we can see that there are many different types of Excedrin®. Excedrin® and Excedrin® Migraine made close to $200 million in sales in 2019. Alternatively, Advil® generated $449.5 million in sales in 2019. Don't just trust my opinion—these hard sales figures demonstrate how others profit from your pain.[1]

The fact that the same drug is marketed to you under a different label happens all the time. One must ask whether this is meant to distinguish brands or just to fool the consumer. Zyban® and Wellbutrin® are actually the same drug, but if you do a Google search for these medicines, you will find it next to impossible to find any sources that reveal they are the same substance. One is marketed to smokers as an anti-smoking drug, while the other is recommended as a treatment for depression.

This marketing is so powerful and pervasive that we are persuaded to think we need to have both types of Excedrin® in our medicine cabinet when they are, in fact, exactly the same medication. We have been taught that a prescription or over-the-counter drug is the solution to all our problems. You've seen all the commercials. There are cute, dancing cartoon characters who go along with each symptom. For stomachache and diarrhea, there's a dance. The rather unattractive, common toe fungus has also been turned into an adorable cartoon character. What kind of fools do these commercial advertisers take us for? I would reply, "Big fools!"

Low Back Pain (LBP)

Most adults have experienced LBP at some point in their lives and either may be experiencing it right now or will do so in the future. There are several different types of LBP (see details in Chapter 9). The standard treatments and recommendations for this condition include hot and cold packs, physical activity, physical therapy, anti-inflammatory medications (like Motrin® or Advil®), and prescription pain pills. Some patients improve, but how many can say their chronic LBP is fully resolved by conventional treatments?

Let's say, for example, you leaned down to pick up something, and *wham!*—you threw your back out. You can barely move now as a result, so you go to see your physician. He prescribes all the therapies I just covered, but nothing really seems to help. So, you go back to your doctor, who now prescribes stronger pain medications and refers you for X-rays, which turn out negative for any significant anatomical damage.

The more potent medications are only a temporary fix, and the pain comes back as soon as the pill wears off. You go back a third time to the doctor. This time, she prescribes physical therapy and sends you out for magnetic resonance imaging (MRI), which looks for soft-tissue damage like pinched nerves or slipped discs. At this point, you have had the pain for three or more months without much relief and are now labeled as a "chronic pain sufferer."

Think about all the people you had to see for your pain: the pharmacist each time you went to get a new pain pill prescription; the physical therapist;

the doctor; and the radiology department personnel for your X-rays and MRI. Let's face it—that's a rather large payroll that is supported by just your pain! Remember what I said about following the money? If your pain were to get better for good, how would all these people earn a living? *The system needs you to continue to be a chronic LBP sufferer.*

In 2021, Big Pharma spent $5.8 billion in direct-to-consumer advertising in the United States.[2] According to the *Washington Post* and Statista, overall pharmaceutical spending on sales and marketing—an enormous $6.58 billion—far outpaces investment in research and development and is only increasing every year.[3] It is not surprising that three of the most frequently advertised medicines are for pain or arthritis: Humira®, Lyrica®, and Xeljanz®. Yet none of these drugs promise total relief.

Let's say you go to CVS Pharmacy or Rite Aid Pharmacy and walk down the pain relief aisle. You'll find signage showing all the medications that will help you fix your LBP. But this is only part of the sell. Even if you originally went to pick up another item, just seeing that sign will prompt your subconscious to say, "Well, my back does hurt—maybe I should buy something I haven't tried yet?" You've just been bribed and will spend money on what is a placeholder treatment at best and won't likely resolve your pain permanently. In contrast, I have seen results that have shown both my patients and me that it doesn't have to be this way.

If you ever wondered why pharmaceutical drugs are so expensive, now you have your answer. With so much money spent on advertising to reinforce the conditioning that leads to that buying decision, those costs have to be assumed by someone. Guess who? Those costs are transferred to us, the unwitting consumers. In effect, we are paying as a society to bribe ourselves!

Television commercials for pharmaceuticals cost a whopping $4.58 billion in 2020. The companies behind these product messages literally buy their way into our lives as a credible go-to source for ailments. And it's best not to ignore the fast-talking pitch person at the end of the commercial who runs down all the possible side effects, which can even include death. No one wants to hear that the remedy for our pain may have horrible side effects or be potentially lethal—so, at your own peril, don't ignore that disclaimer.

You might ask, "Why is that disclaimer sped up so quickly at the tail end of the commercial and difficult to understand?" It seems to be included almost as an afterthought. The marketers want you to focus on the cartoon character or the happy lifestyle scenario of the "cured" person who appears to have gotten her life back after taking "a pill." If you really listened to that fast-talking guy at the end of the commercial as he listed off incontinence, strokes, and other possible side effects, I bet you wouldn't rely on prescription drugs as much.

The Journey to Pain Relief

I regularly see patients who are devastated by their chronic pain. They are so desperate that they are willing to try just about anything I have to offer. After treating thousands of patients who have enjoyed mostly successful outcomes, I can say this with confidence: *You don't need to let another day go by with pain.*

Keep in mind that my patients are achieving pain relief without the need for pain medications or other potentially helpful therapies such as psychotherapy or cognitive behavioral therapy (CBT). That stated, I have nothing against CBT, Tai Chi, or other similar modalities and believe they have value. My aim is to assist you in getting pain free as quickly as possible and without compromising your safety. I have learned firsthand from my patients that when you are pain free, you can get your life back. For many of them, once they are pain free, they often forget what life was like when they were in so much pain.

My focus on this goal started in 2014 when I learned about several game-changing treatments. The first one, which was originally developed in Europe, has some versions that are FDA approved. The second and third are German-based treatments. All three of these modalities have published, peer-reviewed research that demonstrates both their safety and efficacy (see Endnotes). Over the years, I have continued to expand my expertise about these treatments by attending workshops in the United States and Europe. Every day that I am able to help resolve someone's pain, I remember the more than fifty million Americans who are suffering because of profit-driven healthcare and who are, unfortunately, unaware of these proven treatments.

Until we take control of our health and seek to educate ourselves, we will continue to remain victims of a dysfunctional healthcare system. The opioid epidemic is the latest example of how the prescription route has proven to be catastrophic and, in the case of opioids, is specifically due to the overprescribing of pain medications. Thousands have lost their lives as a result of overdoses[4] and thousands more have become addicted to opioid pain medications. The epidemic has occurred despite the fact that pain specialists agree narcotic pain medications are not adequate for pain management. Pain medications are a band-aid. I implore you not to settle for what your doctor or drug advertisers may tell you.

In the chapters that follow, I will be describing the above-mentioned, pioneering modalities for pain relief called pulsed electromagnetic field (PEMF) therapy, neural trigger point therapy, and oxygen-ozone therapy. These are the three treatments that I collectively call The Golden Triad for Pain Relief; they represent the practical key to my mission statement, "You can be pain free."

As these complementary and alternative pain treatments become more well known, it is my hope that patients will ask their doctors to use them. Hopefully, more doctors will also want to learn about them. In the chapters ahead, I will discuss the specific medical conditions that I have treated successfully using these different modalities, and I will also include sections on the role of diet and exercise as well as platelet-rich plasma (PRP) and stem cell therapies.

CHAPTER 3

Eliminating Pain Through Diet

"The journey of a thousand miles begins with a single step."
—Lao Tzu

The role of diet is vital in my practice, and it is an underlying principle for the successful management of pain. My Master of Public Health degree in nutrition from UCLA is foundational to my role as a physician. When a pain patient of mine who has experienced success comes in for a follow-up visit and reports that he'd been doing well, but then suddenly went down-hill, the first question I ask is, "What have you been eating lately?" Almost always with patients like this, the truth comes out that they are making poor food choices.

For some patients, a single dietary infraction can send them spiraling back down into pain for days or weeks. I always try to reassure them that they can come in for pain treatments whenever needed. But I also reinforce their understanding that pain and inflammation are especially responsive to proper diet and nutrition. Poor food choices can cause inflammation, and inflammation can lead to pain.

The Anti-Inflammatory Diet

In particular, what is now called the "gut-brain axis"[1] is talked about extensively in the medical literature.[2] The theory that an anti-inflammatory diet may be beneficial to the gut or the gastrointestinal (GI) microbiome (bacteria in the GI tract) is gaining a lot of traction. This trend supports my initial approach to counseling patients about implementing a pain-preventative diet.[3]

The three most inflammatory foods or food components I ask patients to remove from their diet are gluten, dairy, and sugar.[4] A successful combination I recommend is for them to follow an organic, non-GMO (non-genetically modified organism or pesticide-free foods) regimen, while also avoiding corn and soy. This is supported by a focus on eating a heavily plant-based,[5] low-carbohydrate diet. I emphasize again: if you are suffering from pain and no doctor has yet to suggest a dietary change, you should start by eliminating gluten,[6] dairy, and sugar. Gluten is a protein found in the following grains: wheat, spelt, rye, kamut, and oats (unless specified as gluten free). There are many healthful, delicious, readily available alternative foods that can help you make successful dietary changes in your life. (See some suggested resources in the appendices to this book).

Dr. Hong Shen, a pain management specialist affiliated with the Cleveland Clinic, addresses an elimination diet for neck and back pain, fibromyalgia, and complex regional pain syndrome (pain that lingers after an injury). On the Cleveland Clinic website, she discusses the same diet I mention above.[7]

The Mediterranean diet is another approach to eating which has been recognized for having positive effects including on rheumatoid arthritis. Patients who followed the Mediterranean diet showed a moderate or better clinical improvement in their symptoms versus those who didn't. Also, its beneficial effects on rheumatoid arthritis have been shown in the healthier fats of dieters and as indicated by both the dietary assessment and through the measurement of the blood.[8]

I recognize that changing diets is one of the most difficult things a person can do, so you should know that it doesn't have to be immediate. You can begin gradually. Following this simple plan should bring you some preliminary pain relief. You might find that you do not even need to find a PEMF, neural trigger point, or oxygen-ozone therapy provider.

The Allergy Elimination Diet

For patients who I suspect may have allergies or food sensitivities, I order the IgE test (immunoglobulin E test, measuring true food allergies) and the IgG test (immunoglobulin G test, measuring food sensitivities). When the patient sees she has either food allergy (has IgE positive foods) or food sensitivity or intolerance (IgG positive foods), I have the patient immediately eliminate or rotate these foods. The results can be phenomenal.

A 2019 study published in the journal *Pain Research & Management* demonstrated that an IgG elimination diet as combined with probiotics might be beneficial in both migraine and irritable bowel syndrome (IBS) patients.[9] If you have a history of food allergies or intolerance, ask your doctor to check your blood for these IgG and IgE food antibodies so that you can eliminate them and potentially ameliorate your pain.

If you are not able to get this testing done, then simply remove the most common allergenic foods for three weeks. These include dairy, wheat, sugar, citrus fruits (such as lemons, oranges, tangerines, and grapefruits), eggs, caffeine, alcohol, and any food you eat more than three times a week already. I call it the *allergy elimination diet*.[10]

After three weeks of following this diet, if your pain has improved or disappeared, you then want to find the specific culprit. How? You can do this by reintroducing each of the above foods back into your diet. Add one food back into your regimen every twenty-four to forty-eight hours. Eat that particular "suspect" food in large amounts throughout the day for breakfast, lunch, and dinner. If the pain does not return after two days, then remove that previously suspect food and reintroduce another one from the suspect list. The idea is to test and remove foods every one to two days until you have found the culprit. More often than not, you will discover the offending food or drink.

Once you have found the culprit food, then you may safely add back the other previously suspect foods into your regimen that you had removed from your diet for those three weeks. In the case of migraine headaches, sugar tends to be a prime suspect. Don't just take my word for it—try the elimination diet yourself. If no doctor has recommended this diet yet, and if by trying this diet you get pain relief, then you may have just received your money's worth from purchasing this book.

Lose Weight

Losing weight is recommended if you are obese, overweight, or otherwise suffer from excess body fat.[11] If exercise is out of the question due to severe pain or immobility, then changes to the diet must be employed. The elimination or anti-inflammatory diet can sometimes assist with weight loss, but so can a low-carbohydrate or low-glycemic diet. A functional medicine nutritionist can help you. (See the recommended books in the appendices).

Don't let any doctor tell you there is no science behind this recommendation or that it doesn't work. Trust me, it works well—and that is why it's always my first recommendation to pain patients. There is ample scientific evidence to support your potential trial of this diet. *Sadly, a lot of doctors are not informed about the available research, or they are not properly trained to discuss nutritional factors in illness.*

Stop Smoking!

Smoking contributes to chronic pain and may even be an underlying cause of it.[12] I tell all patients who are smokers that they need to quit ASAP in order for me to help them. Whether it is through their own willpower, prescription medications, herbs, or hypnotherapy, there are multiple methods to stop smoking. Like losing weight, it is not easy to kick the smoking addiction, so ask your doctor for help if you need it.

I have seen patients with chronic LBP experience spontaneous resolution or significant reduction of pain after smoking cessation. Smoking is a really dumb thing to do, anyway, given all the overwhelming, decades-old, scientific evidence showing its relationship to the risk of lung cancer and to cardiovascular and other chronic diseases.

Take Your Supplements

Integrative pain specialists recommend taking omega-3 fats in the form of supplements or eating seafood. In addition, vitamin D3 is anti-inflammatory and quite a useful supplement to combat pain.[13] I measure vitamin D levels in all my patients. All too often, they are deficient in this vitamin. This deficiency is related to our indoor lifestyles since many of us need to work inside and don't get enough sunshine as a result. And those folks who are outdoors often use a lot of sunscreen or are wearing far too many layers of clothing to benefit from the sun's rays.

To make vitamin D in your body, you only need your bare skin and the sunshine. However, once you put on sunblock or layers of clothing, you have effectively blocked the body's ability to make the vitamin D. If you would like to make vitamin D without supplementation, you should make a point of spending time out in the sunshine around high noon for about twenty minutes daily to have sufficient levels—and with as few clothes on as possible. Most of us simply don't have the time to do that or are concerned about skin cancer.

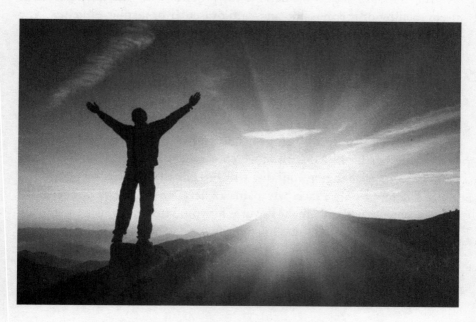

So, I personally resort to and also recommend that my patients take a daily supplement. The recommendations are at least 4,000 IU of vitamin D3 daily taken with food that contains fat. I suggest that you ask your doctor to check for your vitamin D level since it is a standard test now. If your doctor is reluctant for some reason to order the test, then you may safely take 2,000 IU of vitamin D3 daily with a fat-containing meal.

Phytonutrients have been studied and shown to be effective in reducing sickle cell crisis.[14] And rat studies of peripheral neuropathy show benefits of flavonoids in neuropathic pain models.[15]

You Need to Exercise!

Robert Bonakdar, MD, from the Scripps Center for Integrative Medicine stated at the 2018 Pain Care-Primary Care Conference that diet and exercise can bring about a 25 to 30 percent improvement in pain.[16] If you are unable to be physically active, ask your doctor to make out a prescription for physical therapy (PT). Such specialists can design a customized program to get you moving. Taking this step can be life-changing—especially when combined with diet.

The standard recommendations for physical activities are stretching, strengthening of the muscles, and cardiovascular or aerobic exercise.[17] The contrast in the benefits of frequent movement versus inactivity is quite significant when looking at the causes of chronic pain and illness.[18] Physical and mental well-being can improve dramatically with exercise in pain patients. Hatha Yoga and Tai Chi are two very gentle exercise styles you can try (especially the latter). Classes in both are offered online and in person. So, ask your doctor to assist you in your goal to become physically active.

Remember that by just being outside, you are getting sunshine, vitamin D, and the Earth's PEMFs, all of which can help reduce or eliminate your pain. Of course, changing your diet will also greatly help. Eating poorly and being sedentary only exacerbate pain, anxiety, and depression; these two lifestyle choices will only make it worse for you. Finally, if you are a smoker, remember how important it is to stop smoking when attempting to reduce chronic pain.

CHAPTER 4

Pain Therapy That Works:
Pulsed Electromagnetic
Field (PEMF) Therapy

"For every shadow, no matter how deep, is threatened
by morning light."
—*The Fountain (2006)*

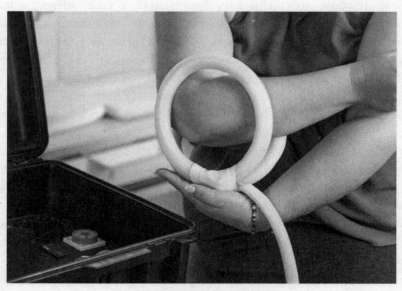

PEMF therapy for elbow pain.

Every new patient who comes into my office with primary or secondary pain symptoms (the pain is not their main reason for seeing me) will get a complimentary session of PEMF therapy. Sometimes the pain is relieved instantaneously and never returns. Quite often, the patient forgets he even had the pain until I ask about it on the subsequent follow-up visit. For many patients, if there is a temporary improvement, I recommend they return for repeat treatments anywhere from one to three times a week for a total of ten sessions to get the full benefits.

PEMF Therapy

Pulsed electromagnetic field therapy, or PEMF therapy, was first developed in Europe in the twentieth century. Since then, it has inspired more than ten thousand publications in the medical literature.[1] More than two thousand double-blind studies have been published.[2] Initial research on the technology was conducted in Russia and Eastern Europe. More recently, expanded research has been performed in the United States. In the 1980s, the FDA approved the first PEMF device for use in the stimulation of bone growth in non-union fractures. By the 1990s, much of Europe had already become familiar with PEMF therapy. Clearly, the safety and efficacy of PEMF therapy has now been established.

PEMF treatments are generally short, cost-efficient, and, according to some studies on osteoarthritis, have eliminated the need for surgery in many cases[3,4] and male pelvic pain[5] syndromes such as endometriosis, ruptured ovarian cysts, and prostatitis showed PEMF therapy as a useful, effective modality. A 2016 paper in the *International Journal of Clinical Trials* concluded: "PEMF (10 Hz, 4-5mT) can be considered as a beneficial and persistent prophylactic treatment option for refractory migraine."[6]

Other conditions that benefit from PEMF therapy include fibromyalgia,[7] diabetic polyneuropathy,[8] LBP,[9] and osteoarthritis.[10,11] The results are often seen quickly. In one study of patients with disc herniation, anxiety, and depression, their pain and quality of life improved with PEMF therapy.[12] Very early on in this book I talked about how anxiety, depression, insomnia, and poor quality of life accompany chronic pain. PEMF therapy has the potential to help with all of these symptoms. A paper published in 2007 talked about the benefits of PEMF therapy for migraine headaches.[13] [14] Sadly, most doctors are not yet aware of this.

PEMF therapy also appears to be beneficial for more than just pain. I've observed it to be useful for the following conditions: improvement of immune function, speedier healing of skin wounds, reduction of inflammation and swelling, improvement of sleep, enhancement of bone health (osteoporosis), and regeneration of nerve tissue.

Transcranial magnetic stimulation is another form of PEMF therapy that is FDA approved for the treatment of psychiatric disorders such as depression. Two thousand randomized clinical trials and ten thousand publications later, PEMF therapy has been demonstrated to be safe and efficacious; yet, regrettably, it's still not an accepted mainstream treatment. This may be one reason your doctor didn't tell you about PEMF therapy.

One explanation is that randomized clinical trials to date have not included large enough patient numbers (high-powered studies), so they are not regarded as adequate. PEMF therapy is an effective treatment for many medical conditions, especially pain.[15] Another explanation is that since it's not a patentable pharmaceutical drug, PEMF therapy does not represent the same kind of significant corporate profit center.

How Does PEMF Therapy Work?

How does PEMF therapy eliminate pain? The answer is multifactorial. PEMF therapy uses a device that generates an electrical current to modify the pain signal coming from your brain. The device does this by applying an electromagnetic field to the affected area. When your cells are unhealthy due to disease or inflammation, the electrical voltage of the specific cells is lower. PEMF therapy works to restore your cells to their normal electrical membrane potential. By doing so, PEMF therapy eliminates or significantly reduces pain.[16] PEMF therapy also can heal injury or trauma.[17,18,19]

Often, I hear patients confusing transcutaneous electrical nerve stimulation (TENS) therapy with pulsed electromagnetic field (PEMF) therapy. There is a difference between the two treatments.[20] TENS is more of an electrical stimulation, while PEMF therapy uses a magnetic field to treat the pain. I find PEMF therapy far more effective than TENS.

Since your body is made up of mostly water, PEMF therapy will oxygenate, alkalinize, and hydrate your cells, with the result that the transfer of nutrients across your cell membranes will be improved. Ultimately, it can enhance energy production and resolve your pain (see footnote 16). Bryant A. Meyers explains in his book *PEMF* how the Earth's magnetic fields are just as essential for life and survival as food, water, sunlight, and oxygen. The Earth's PEMFs protect us from the harmful radiation of the sun. In a certain sense, the cause of disease can be explained as a disconnection of our own bodies from the earth's PEMFs.

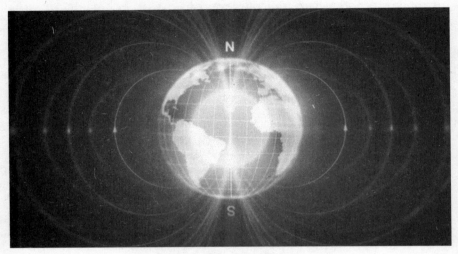

Example of Earth's PEMFs.

Many of us spend most of our day indoors and away from direct sunlight, the earth's PEMFs, and fresh air. We also can be guilty of failing to eat healthful, whole foods and not hydrating adequately. Earth-based PEMF machines that operate at frequencies similar to the frequency of the human body are the machines that have been studied the most for pain. The hypothesis behind their effectiveness is that the low frequency produced by PEMF machines resonates with that of our own cells. The procedure can help restore the proper functioning of our cells, which alleviates the pain. Treatment duration can be several minutes up to thirty minutes, twice daily for many days or weeks before realizing benefits.

If you read nothing further in this book, you can do just one thing for yourself if you are a chronic pain sufferer, and it's quite simple: try to spend at least one hour a day outdoors, barefoot if possible, so that you can benefit from Mother Nature's natural PEMFs. This is similar to grounding mats but the PEMF from the earth is more powerful.

The PEMF machine I utilize in my office is the opposite of this low frequency type. Instead, it is potent in intensity and is applied to the area of pain for a very brief period, where it can bring almost instant pain relief. The PEMF coils are placed on the affected area of the body and are left in place while the machine emits an electromagnetic current to the cells and tissues. The PEMF stays on that same area of the body for just a few minutes.

As I write this chapter on PEMF, I am experimenting with the low frequency, Earth-based-type PEMF to see if it might benefit those patients who didn't have success from the more powerful version. I respectfully disagree with Bryant Meyers, an author and expert in the field of PEMF, who advises against trying the high-intensity PEMF machines. Having used one on my patients for six years now, I can say it is safe and instrumental in pain resolution.

So, there are currently two options when choosing which PEMF machine to try. If you try one type first—say the low-frequency PEMF machine—and it doesn't bring you pain relief, then be sure to try the high-intensity PEMF machine, which just might do the trick. Regardless of the type of PEMF machine you are using, it really helps to drink two glasses of water thirty minutes prior to treatment to get the best results.

Let's now look at several typical cases where I found PEMF therapy to have been especially effective.

Ryan's Story: Chronic Neck/Back Pain and PEMF Therapy

Ryan is a forty-nine-year-old male who suffered with chronic LBP that began when he was a teenager and wrestled in high school and college. At that time, he was diagnosed with arthritis of the back. Subsequently, thirteen years ago, he was rear-ended and has since developed chronic neck pain accompanied with stiffness. He was told that the diagnosis was osteoarthritis. After the first PEMF treatment, Ryan noticed it helped both his neck and LBP. He has come back and done at least ten sessions of PEMF therapy. The treatment has made a huge difference in allowing him to continue his active lifestyle.

Larry's Story: Chronic Neck Pain and PEMF Therapy

Larry is a forty-five-year-old male who had sustained a neck injury (cervical spine) four months before I saw him. He was given cortisone injections and traction therapy under his former doctor, neither of which helped manage his pain. While under that doctor's care, he had also become dangerously dependent on painkillers. His initial purpose for seeing me was for oxygen-ozone injections. However, I like to suggest starting with PEMF therapy first, and after just one session, he no longer was experiencing any neck pain. In addition, he was able to sleep for twelve hours straight, which he had not been able to do since the injury. His tightness and numbness also improved as a result of treatment. Needless to say, he didn't require the oxygen-ozone injections from me.

Nina's Story: Chronic Body Aches, Joint Pain, and PEMF Therapy

Nina is a seventy-two-year-old female who presented with generalized body aches, including right shoulder pain due to osteoarthritis, chronic neck pain, and joint stiffness. Just one PEMF treatment took away her muscle aches for an entire week. When I saw her on a follow-up appointment a month later, she had not done any further PEMF therapy, but she stated she was not in as much pain as before.

Valerie's Story: Rheumatoid Arthritis and PEMF Therapy

Valerie is a sixty-four-year-old female who is suffering from rheumatoid arthritis, resulting in symptoms of chronic shoulder pain and chronic knee pain. After her second PEMF session, she noticed a significant improvement in her knee pain. While I still had to treat her shoulder pain with oxygen-ozone injections, her knees have not bothered her since the original series of ten PEMF treatments, which was about four years ago.

Is PEMF Therapy a Consideration for You?

It's important to note the patients for whom PEMF therapy is contraindicated: it is not recommended for patients who are pregnant, have seizure disorder, or wear implantable pacemakers. Aside from these exceptions, anyone can try PEMF therapy.

If my patient does not respond to PEMF therapy, I recommend two other fantastic treatment modalities for pain—neural trigger point therapy and oxygen-ozone therapy. After reading this chapter and knowing that there are thousands of research articles on PEMF therapy, don't you think everyone with pain ought to get a trial treatment? It is non-invasive, non-pharmacological, and almost always without any adverse effects. As stated earlier, a version of PEMF therapy has been approved by the FDA for the treatment of depression and nonunion joint fracture. A number of my patients express improvement in their depression and anxiety from PEMF therapy. PEMF provides another reason to have hope of being free from anxiety and depression and returning to work and productivity.

CHAPTER 5

The "Queen" of Pain Relief:
Neural Trigger Point Therapy

"You need something to open up a new door,
to show you something you seen before but overlooked a
hundred times or more."

—Bob Dylan

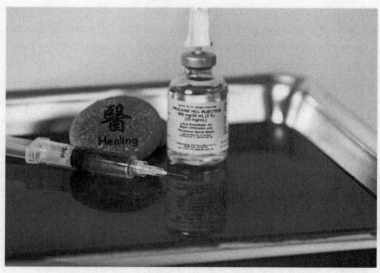

Bottle of Novocain and syringe with small needle for almost all
neural trigger point therapy injections.

Janet Travell, MD, was the White House physician under former presidents John F. Kennedy and Lyndon B. Johnson. Kennedy suffered greatly from chronic LBP. Dr. Travell was an expert in treating myofascial inflammation and pain.[1] Myofascial relates to fascia, a thin sheath of tissue that surrounds and separates muscle tissue. She is said to have traveled to Germany to learn neural trigger point therapy. However, it is believed that she only brought back a single aspect of the technology, and as a result, became known as the founder and the "Trigger Queen"[2] of trigger point injection therapy. Had she utilized all the principles of neural trigger point therapy, this treatment strategy would be a medical mainstay today, and primary care doctors like myself would be successfully using it to treat pain on a daily basis. In the pages that follow, I am going to explain to you why I believe "the Queen" missed the boat on this one.

Pain and the Lymphatic System

Every patient gets a regular physical and a neural trigger point therapy exam before they receive any treatment in my office. The examination involves looking for pain in areas where most doctors don't think to look. It's my belief that the lymphatic system is involved in the genesis of pain for some patients. If I find tenderness on palpation (feeling with my fingers) in the inguinal (groin) region, I perform the neural trigger point therapy in that area. Quite often, any pain in the legs, shins, feet, or ankles may disappear immediately.

The likely explanation here is that the lymphatic system connects to the nervous system and is a source of energy blockage. Neural trigger point therapy appears to restore this flow of energy through the nerves and lymphatics. The physical exam also involves pressing over the peri-axillary region (next to the armpit), groin, shins, and neck muscles (trapezius region). If the trapezius is tender, it indicates tonsillar involvement which requires injections in that area, (see Rain's story later in this chapter).

Interestingly, Bryan L. Frank, MD, noted the connection between the lymphatics and pain in his article titled "Neural Therapy": "In the 1970s, Fleckenstein (father of Calcium Antagonism and professor of physiology and pharmacology) showed that the injection of Novocain into lymphatic vessels or nodes led to the dilation of the lymphatic vessels and increased the speed of transport of lymph through the entire lymphatic system. Chronic spasm of the lymphatics may exist for long periods from injury or illness, and local anesthetic injections likely open the channels and resume normal lymphatic flow."[3] (See additional resources in the appendices.)

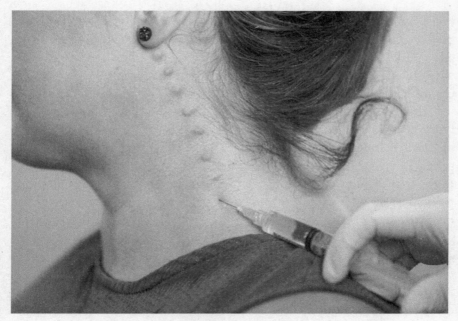

Example of what neural trigger point therapy blebs look like.

As an experiment, try pressing over your groin, armpit area, and shins to find any tenderness or pain on yourself. If it is present, and you have some chronic pain complaint in and around that area, then you may benefit from neural trigger point therapy.

As another example, many patients with foot or ankle pain complaints will find their pain gone once I have injected their groin region with these tiny blebs of procaine. I can bring about pain relief by treating only the lymphatic area for possible blockage without needing to treat the actual location of the pain.

Energy Blockage and Flow

First of all, the best thing about neural trigger point therapy is that if it doesn't work, it didn't do any harm. Neural trigger point therapy is based on the theory that any trauma, infection, or surgery can damage the autonomic nervous system and produce long-standing disturbances in the electrochemical or electromagnetic functions of tissues. It was developed in the early twentieth century by Drs. Ferdinand and Walter Huneke, who were brothers and physicians practicing in Germany. They had an understanding of Chinese medicine and the concept of the flow of "Chi" energy in the body. Ayurvedic medicine, which is still practiced in India and Pakistan, predates Chinese medicine by several thousand years. Ayurvedic medicine also speaks to the "Prana" or life force energy. Both traditions agree that when there is blockage of the flow of energy (stagnation), there will be disease or pathology.

There are many examples in modern medicine that demonstrate how humans are energy-conducting beings, yet this has yet to be translated into medical treatments. The electrocardiogram (ECG) and electroencephalogram (EEG) measure the electrical current of the heart and brain, respectively, and demonstrate that the body is an electric field. Neural trigger point therapy offers a way to directly impact the electrical energy of the human body.

The Neural Trigger Point Therapy Breakthrough

Neural trigger point therapy was shown in one study to be the "stronger cousin" of acupuncture,[4] and it follows many of the same time-tested principles mentioned above. It does use the anesthetic Novocain (which is also known by the generic drug name of procaine), to achieve sometimes miraculous results when it comes to pain.

I know what you might be thinking at this point: "What is she talking about Novocain and procaine are pharmaceutical drugs, which this writer was criticizing in an earlier chapter!" Actually, the anesthetic Novocain has been around for about a hundred years and has a long track record of safety. More importantly, it is not mass-produced because it is not a real money maker. It has been largely replaced by newer, longer-acting dental anesthetics. Also, it must be made by compounding pharmacies for doctors like myself. If a patient has an aversion to using Novocain, then I am also able to get the same results using sterile saline. I have often wondered if Procaine/Novocain can be replaced with saline exclusively. No one has yet studied this possibility formally.

Drs. Ferdinand and Walter Huneke discovered that just as in Chinese medicine, there are what they called *interference fields*. These are local tissue irritations, scars, areas of trauma, or areas of stagnation in the body that can accumulate toxins or disturb energetic flow. The same is true when discussing an application for neural trigger point therapy. Believe it or not, the area that this occurs in first and foremost is your tonsils—yes, the tonsils! Most of us have had infections that affect the throat—viral infections like infectious mononucleosis and Epstein-Barr virus, or bacterial infections like streptococcal pharyngitis (more commonly known as strep throat). If you are older like me, then you most likely had chickenpox or measles (vaccines weren't available for these two when I was little). All these infections attack your tonsils.

When a patient who has a prior history of these infections comes to me with neck or jaw pain, I inject a small amount of procaine just above and below each tonsil. The patient may then experience a complete resolution of the neck or jaw pain. You might be somewhat skeptical and are thinking, "Wait a minute! If you are injecting an anesthetic, shouldn't the area injected get numb and be pain free because of that?"

Yes, you are correct. Procaine and its metabolites (molecules from the procaine itself breaking down) break down quickly. It follows that if your theory is correct, then the pain should return once the anesthetic has worn off. However, in many cases it doesn't return immediately. Once the patient has experienced relief following the tonsillar injections, pain can come back—but days or a week later. This indicates the patient needs to return to have a few more sessions of the tonsillar injections to become permanently pain free.

The main contraindication to neural trigger point therapy is an allergy to procaine or similar anesthetics. However, using sterile saline instead of procaine can give you just about the same results. Drs. Walter and Ferdinand Huneke were well aware of this factor and discussed it in their writings. Even if you are not a fan of getting injected with an anesthetic, you can try the saline alternative of neural trigger point therapy.

Rain's Story: Tonsillar Injections, Neural Trigger Point Therapy, and Chronic Pain

"Dr. Hirani is giving me my life back. Maybe that sounds a bit dramatic, but it is true. I've been living with chronic illness for over twenty years now. I'd been deteriorating for this long because other doctors either minimized my issues or just didn't know what to do to help or weren't interested in trying. My mom found Dr. Hirani over a year ago, but I was reluctant to come because of my past experiences.

"When I first saw her, she said, 'We're going to try to get to the bottom of this, and I won't tell you it's all in your head,' and I literally cried in her office. A little spark of hope was rekindled in me. I still had pessimism so as not to get my hopes dashed again. She took an incredibly detailed history, way more than any other doctor I had seen did. She took the time to listen to my story, and that is not what I had been used to. Chronic fatigue syndrome was my primary diagnosis before going to see Dr. Hirani, and it kept me homebound.

"When I started the neural trigger point therapy, I didn't realize how much my pain was contributing to my illness. Sure, I was achy and uncomfortable and got worse with weather changes. But the neural trigger point therapy started to take it away. She told me to go gluten free, and within two weeks, I noticed that my pain got even better. For years, I had trouble lying on my sides to sleep at night due to pain, which was now going away.

"The neural trigger point therapy involved a series of neural trigger point injections all over my body. They are painful for me as I have a low threshold for pain, but what was amazing after a day or two was how much less the pain was. The tonsillar injections took away my chronic shoulder-neck pain with 'knots' completely! My husband, who massages me there, even noticed that the knots were gone, and the area was no longer painful with the massage.

"She treated my endometriosis and adenomyosis as well as my migraines with neural therapy. One day, I was experiencing a migraine at my appointment with Dr. Hirani. The neural IV procaine push took it away almost immediately. Now if I get a migraine, I am not bedbound like I used to be for one to three days. I can just rest, then I can function around the house.

"I have continued with regular neural trigger point therapy treatments. My pain continues to diminish, and my chronic fatigue, which I had gone to see Dr. Hirani for, has also improved tremendously. She has done specific functional medical tests and has corrected nutritional deficiencies and hormonal imbalances in me, which have also contributed to my successful path toward healing."

My patient Rain, who suffered with chronic tender knots over her trapezius muscles, was in disbelief when her pain and knots instantly disappeared after the tonsillar injections. I've seen that jaw pain can be relieved in the same way for many patients. Just how many times a patient needs a repeat injection depends on the individual. I advise four to six injection sessions about every one to two weeks. I caution the patient to expect that some injection site soreness may last typically for an hour or two, after which it spontaneously resolves. Only rarely does it last a couple days. Either way, I explain it's no big deal if the pain lasts a little longer, taking into consideration the anticipated results.

The depth of the injection is only several millimeters, so it is considered minimally invasive. I use this injection in my chronic fatigue patients, who often experience tremendous relief from the associated fatigue. If you suffer from chronic pain in the head, neck, or jaw region, you owe it to yourself to try this treatment. It is a minor procedure compared to the deep injections your dentist gives you to numb your mouth prior to dental work. If you have chronic pain anywhere with an accompanying fatigue factor, then this is the appropriate injection for you to request from a trained neural trigger point therapy doctor.

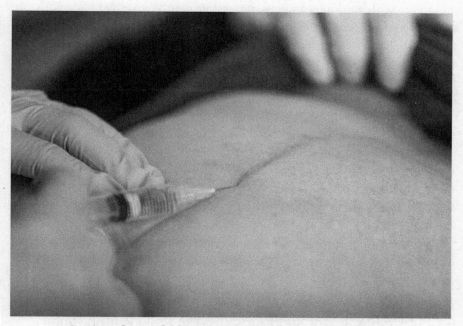

Scar/interference field injection in neural trigger point therapy.

Scars and surgical or traumatic injuries (these days, even from piercings such as belly button rings and tattoos) are another considerable interference field. These can also be causes of chronic pain. Eliminating the interference field due to scars is probably the most effortless injection for doctors to perform and the easiest one for patients to receive. Injecting just under the scar and along its entire length with the smallest amount of procaine is all it takes. It is a tiny, half-inch, 30-gauge needle.

Neural trigger-point therapy has the potential to bring about an emotional release while improving symptoms of pain or chronic illness like chronic fatigue.[5] Some patients may have a crying episode or feelings of sadness that give way to feelings of joy and calmness. Although it is not a usual occurrence, it is welcomed when it does happen.

Billie's Story: Neural Trigger Point Therapy Scar Treatment

Billie was a former Vidal Sassoon model. She suffered from chronic neck pain as a result of two surgeries performed for cosmetic purposes and ended up disabled.

Visits with multiple doctors, including neurologists, left her with no answers and only pain pill prescriptions. She was unable to drive or work and had become dependent on these medications. When she came to me, she sounded hopeless. I promised her that if the scar injections along the back of her neck were going to work, it would be instantaneous. As I predicted, within minutes of my being finished, she was pain free.

She was able to move her neck around and no longer had a limited range of motion. Billie was in disbelief. She had been suffering for so long, and no one had told her that she could get rid of her pain with injections into her plastic surgery scars. I'm happy that Billie is another patient of mine who got her life back again.

She started driving, grocery shopping, and resumed her once normal, active life. Also, she never needed to repeat those injections after that first time. So, if you or someone you know is a chronic pain sufferer with scars, it is imperative to determine if these scars are, in fact, interference fields by trying the neural trigger point therapy injection route.

From Irritable Bowel Syndrome (IBS) to Belly Button Rings

I can't tell you the number of times I've seen the connection between IBS and belly button piercing in women. A previous piercing over the belly button can contribute to IBS. This is a condition accompanied by abdominal pain that alternates with diarrhea or loose stools and constipation. Anxiety is another common symptom these patients have. Merely injecting the belly button scar, tattoo (located in the area of IBS pain), cesarean section or appendectomy scar can bring about pain relief. It can also result in the elimination of nervousness—and again, the results are often instantaneous.

As previously mentioned in Rain's story, the tonsils are a significant interference field, but the tonsillectomy scar is also a huge interference field.

Patients with previous tonsillectomies who present with pain in the head or neck region usually don't know that the pain could be due to this scar. The injection is similar to other scar injections in that it is very superficial and made along the length of the scar at the back of the throat. Quite often, the scar is visible to the naked eye. You can use your mirror and shine a bright light into your open mouth to see that white scar at the back of your throat from a previous tonsillectomy.

The Sinuses

The sinuses are the third interference field found in neural trigger point therapy. Many patients with headaches or chronic sinus congestion and pain are likely candidates for this treatment. As long as a patient presents with a history of sinus problems and/or sinus headaches—regardless of where their primary pain problem lies—a sinus pattern is indicated. The treatment will entail a series of blebs made with a half-inch needle just under the surface of the skin (intradermal). Again, a small volume of procaine is injected into each site. It is performed over acupuncture points on the face using procaine. I've found the results to be exceptional. (See Chapter 8 for illustration of the sinus pattern neural trigger point therapy blebs).

The Trigger Points

Once the interference fields are treated and eliminated, then localized injections over the area of pain (trigger point) is a primary goal in neural trigger point therapy. This is analogous to the trigger point injections that former President John F. Kennedy's White House staff physician, Dr. Janet Travell, taught. However, they are not intramuscular (like Dr. Travell's injections); instead, they are the same superficial blebs I perform right over the area of pain, sometimes followed by a subcutaneous injection of procaine.

Danny's Story: Multiple Sclerosis (MS) Pain and
Neural Trigger Point Therapy

Danny is a patient who regularly comes in for neural trigger point therapy treatments. She suffers from MS and has chronic pain in many parts of her body. When she first came to me, she was crying due to her pain and weakness in her legs. She believed she was going to be a cripple soon and be completely unable to walk.

I simply performed several dozen blebs of procaine over the tender spots along her thighs, which included the sides, inner, and front portions. When she left the office, she was pain free and able to walk with increased strength—and without the help of a cane! She has since come to me to have similar treatments done to her arms, neck, and sacral (buttock) area monthly—each time with immediate results. Like the previous case of Billie, she has been able to reclaim her life and attributes this success exclusively to neural trigger point therapy.

Neural Trigger Point Therapy Is Here to Stay

Neural trigger point therapy has been practiced in many countries since 1920, but it is still relatively unknown in the United States. Hundreds, if not thousands, of published papers exist on its benefits and safety. Publications include studies of the following areas and issues for which it has been shown to be effective: pelvic pain in women, MS, urodynamic bladder,[6] chronic LBP, and chronic pain in general.[7,8]

Dietrich Klinghardt, MD, PhD, a German physician, is credited for bringing the practice of neural trigger point therapy from Europe to the United States. Like many other practitioners, I have benefitted from his contributions to the field, and as a result, so have my patients. Robert F. Kidd, MD, CM, also wrote a useful book on neural therapy for practitioners titled *Neural Therapy: Applied Neurophysiology and Other Topics.*[9]

The "Queen" of Pain Treatments

I am not the only doctor who has witnessed dramatic improvements in patients' pain using neural trigger point therapy, and I am glad it is getting more attention from the medical community in the United States. American doctors like Tracy Brobyn, MD, have published articles on neural trigger point therapy. She has stated: "Our center has witnessed numerous cases where this technique has led to dramatic improvement and often complete cure of a patient's long-term pain."[10]

From my point of view, another benefit is that consultations required for treatment are short. Even better, possible adverse effects are next to none. Many of my patients reduce or eliminate their need for chronic pain medications as a result of this treatment. Neural trigger point therapy is also cost-effective and practical—especially when you add in the benefits of quality of life, happiness, and ability to function and work. An added side benefit of neural trigger point therapy is that it seems to help with anxiety as it is resetting the nervous system when performed correctly. This aspect of neural trigger point therapy represents an added benefit to patients suffering from anxiety because of their pain condition.

The only contraindications to neural trigger point therapy are an allergy to procaine (Novocain), at the site of an active cancer or infection, pregnancy, or severe psychological instability (due to the kind of emotional release that can sometimes ensue after treatment—see footnote 5).

I refer to neural trigger point therapy as the "Queen" of pain treatments. But when neural trigger point therapy is not successful in bringing my patients relief, I utilize another advanced tool from The Golden Triad for Pain Relief—oxygen-ozone therapy.

CHAPTER 6

The "King" of Pain Relief:
Oxygen-Ozone Therapy

"If you reveal your secrets to the wind,
you should not blame the wind for revealing them to the trees."
—Khalil Gibran

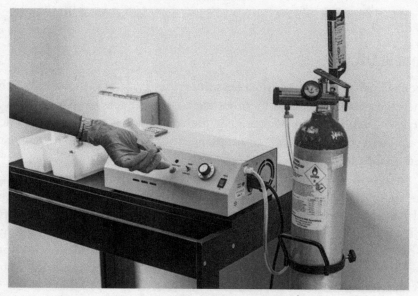

Ozone gas being generated in the syringe prior to treatment.

About 30,000 practitioners of oxygen-ozone therapy exist in the world today. Germany has the most significant number with more than 11,000 doctors. China is next with 5,000. Russia comes up third with 3,500, followed by Italy with 3,000 doctors. The exact number of United States doctors practicing oxygen-ozone therapy is not known, but this country clearly lags behind the other forward-thinking countries, and I hope to see that number change rapidly.

More than three thousand articles have been published on medical oxygen-ozone therapy, especially as focused on the subject of LBP and spinal disc disease. It is now an accepted form of medical treatment in twelve countries. Russia has been conducting animal and human studies on oxygen-ozone for more than fifty years. In Germany, it has been estimated that around ten million treatments of oxygen-ozone therapy have been performed to date. At this stage, its safety and efficacy are undisputed.

First of all, when applied in therapeutic or low doses, oxygen-ozone does not harm normal, healthy cells. It makes your blood more fluid, strengthens the immune system, is anti-inflammatory, and, most importantly for my practice, it is analgesic (a pain reliever).[1,2] Oxygen-ozone helps your cells produce your own antioxidants,[3] stimulates the creation of cytokines (chemical messengers) to reduce inflammation, boosts the immune system, and gets rid of pain.[4] In other words, it can bring profound relief to patients.

What is Ozone?

Ozone is a gas made up of three oxygen molecules. It was discovered in the nineteenth century by the German chemist and professor Dr. Christian Friedrich Schonbein in Switzerland. He coined the term "ozone," which means "bad smell" in Greek. Since then, many different uses of ozone have been applied in medicine.

In World War I, ozone was used by German doctors to treat trench foot in soldiers who had sustained bad infections. Pioneering scientist Nikola Tesla patented the first ozone generator here in the United States in 1896. By the late 1800s, ozone was used to purify water in several countries, such as Russia and Holland. It succeeded in beating typhoid fever in the early 1900s in European cities where it was used for water purification.

In 1904, Charles Marchand, a French chemist who had moved to New York, published a book titled *The Medical Uses of Hydrozone and Glycozone* (ozonated olive oil) in the United States. This book now sits in the Library of Congress with a stamp of approval by the US Surgeon General.[5] Ozone was commonly used by American doctors around the turn of the 1900s when the American Medical Association abruptly removed it—apparently for no good reason. It has never been known to cause any significant harm when used appropriately. Since it is literally made up of oxygen, no one is allergic to ozone, and it doesn't interact with drugs. It only interacts positively with cells and tissues inside the body.

Energized Oxygen

Professor Velio Bocci, an Italian medical doctor and professor of physiology, wrote the 2005 book, *Ozone: A New Medical Drug*,[6] which investigated ozone's effect on white blood cells. His research found that ozone caused them to produce cytokines or chemical messengers that could attack infections. It has been referred to as "energized oxygen" and is a very potent oxidizing agent—and that is precisely why people are afraid of it. However, in small amounts (which is how ozone is meant to be used in medicine), ozone has excellent healing properties that go beyond just that of analgesia (inability to feel pain). Ozone has been used to treat multiple medical conditions from cardiovascular disease to cancer. Promising research shows that it can help regenerate damaged tissue in joints and cartilage.[7]

Michael E. Shannon, MD, the former deputy surgeon general of Canada, has repeatedly spoken of ozone's analgesic effects, including in the 2004 documentary titled *Ozone, a Medical Breakthrough*.[8] This film addresses the various applications of this medical treatment. The documentary explores the real reasons why ozone is not considered a standard of care for the treatment of chronic pain and other illnesses. As stated earlier, more than three thousand research papers exist on its use in medicine. The bottom line is that the medical establishment has no incentive to study it since ozone is not patentable. Thus, oxygen-ozone therapy hasn't received the attention it rightly deserves.

How Does Oxygen-ozone therapy Work?

According to existing research, ozone's mechanism of action in low doses is as follows: It influences your cells to produce antioxidants, antioxidant enzyme systems, and cytokines to reduce inflammation, kill viruses and bacteria, and boost the immune system. In addition, it also shuts off your body's pain receptors when it is administered locally as an injection. For these reasons, oxygen-ozone therapy is a fantastic tool in our practice. As previously mentioned, assuming that the patient has not had success with PEMF therapy or neural trigger point therapy, then the next step is oxygen-ozone therapy.

Once the oxygen-ozone is injected, the pain can be eliminated. There is a reason why I refer to it as the "King" of pain relief—when my other two treatment modalities from The Golden Triad for Pain Relief, PEMF and neural trigger point therapy, don't deliver the results I want for my patients, oxygen-ozone will more than likely come through to save the day.

Intra-articular (direct injection into the joints) injection using oxygen-ozone is excellent for osteoarthritis and joint pain in general.[9] From the cervical spine to the lumbar spine, these injections can eliminate the need for surgery in many people. The same goes for osteoarthritis in the knees, wrists, ankles, shoulders, or hips. In the chapters that follow, I will discuss the specific pain conditions in more detail and how I use oxygen-ozone therapy. You will also read testimonials from ecstatic, pain-free patients.

At the heart of my practice, I derive a lot of pleasure in seeing my patients becoming pain free. On occasion, I have a patient who will take about two weeks before the pain relief happens, so I always alert patients about this possibility.

A simple PubMed® search of "oxygen-ozone and joint pain" produces numerous results. Search results are extensive on Google when exploring the use and effectiveness of oxygen-ozone therapy for various conditions. It is useful in the treatment of rheumatoid arthritis, various back disorders like herniated discs,[10,11,12,13,14] hip bursitis,[15] frozen shoulder,[16] and even temporomandibular joint (TMJ) dysfunction.[17]

My clinical results with these types of patients mirror the research findings. Many European studies show that oxygen-ozone injections for treatment of knee osteoarthritis result in pain relief, the disappearance of edema (swelling), and improved mobility.[18] This "King of pain relief" can be a more effective and safer substitute for the standard medications that are often unsuccessful when prescribed to treat many painful musculoskeletal conditions.

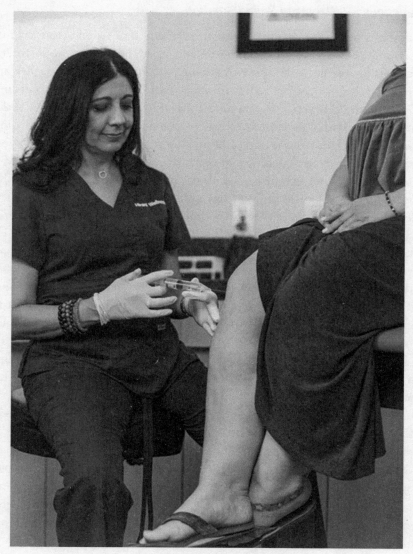

Dr. Hirani injected the knee with ozone.

The following are contraindications for ozone treatment: glucose-6-phosphate dehydrogenase (G6PD) deficiency in patients receiving intravenous ozone-oxygen therapy, hyperthyroidism, thrombocytopenia (platelet disorder), recent heart attack, seizure disorder, and hemorrhagic conditions (bleeding disorders).

Intravenous (IV) Ozonized Saline Solution

Intravenous ozone can be used to treat pain as a stand-alone treatment or in conjunction with other modalities. When a patient is not a candidate for injections (for example, the above treatments were not successful, or they are afraid of injections), then IV saline ozone is what I will prescribe. According to Dr. Adriana Schwartz, "The method consists in the prior saturation of the saline solution with a mixture of oxygen-ozone and its intravenous infusion to the patient. This route of application was approved by the Ministry of Health of the Russian Federation in the early eighties of the last century,"[19] She also says, "The recommended doses of ozone to be used in O3SS [ozonized saline solution] are very low and are calculated by weight of the patient. These have been detailed and endorsed in item 3.1.22 of the Madrid Declaration on Ozone Therapy."[20] Thousands of patients have received IV saline ozone without any major problems. So, it's considered to be safe and potentially very beneficial.

Its primary purpose is to help the body produce plenty of antioxidants that will help reduce inflammation and, consequently, any associated pain. If a patient notices relief of his pain almost instantaneously after the IV saline ozone, then it is the right treatment for them.

For example, I have a patient with chronic headaches and fibromyalgia who regularly comes in for IV saline ozone and PEMF treatments. This patient needs nerve blocks to the cervical spinal nerves when she is not coming to my office regularly. She is still dependent on narcotic pain meds. When she receives the PEMF and the IV saline ozone therapies, it brings down her pain level and gives her more energy.

Even though she has not experienced complete relief with these complementary and alternative pain methods, she keeps coming back for them and is grateful for the relief they provide. She has related how the treatments give her enhanced quality of life, which she doesn't experience regularly with her traditional medical regimen.

CHAPTER 7

Self-Regeneration: Platelet-Rich Plasma (PRP) and Stem Cells for Pain

"Innovation distinguishes between a leader
and a follower."

—Steve Jobs

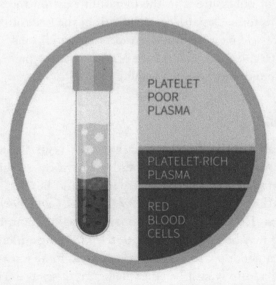

Platelet-Rich Plasma (PRP) derived from the patient's own blood.

I have a patient who lives in Las Vegas and comes to our Los Angeles office approximately every four weeks for PRP/oxygen-ozone injections to both ankles. She has chronic pain after several ankle surgeries on both sides, with accompanying metal plates and screws. She first came in requesting stem cells or biological allograft (explained below), which she received. The second time she came in, we only did PRP and oxygen-ozone therapy, and she saw excellent results. Since then, she comes in asking only for these two treatments for her ankles.

Following her successful treatment, this patient was able to walk all over Europe during her summer vacation. Her pain condition has continued to improve significantly from what it was before the injections. Her quality of life has also improved. Before the PRP/oxygen-ozone injections, she would never have dreamed of walking throughout Europe.

PRP and Your Blood

Platelets in your blood are essential for blood clotting and wound healing. They contain growth factors like stem cells that can aid in reducing inflammation and pain. PRP cell fragments come from your own blood ("autologous" means "to be obtained from the same individual"). After a simple blood draw, a tube of blood is spun down and separates out the red cells. This clear "liquid gold" that is left over is the PRP.

Thousands of publications in the literature exist on the successful use of PRP injections for back pain, osteoarthritis of the knee, ankle and elbow pain, skeletal muscle pain, tendinitis, and other conditions.[1] These studies demonstrate PRP injections can reduce or eliminate the pain and be a safer alternative to steroid injections in the long term.

PRP: Background

PRP therapy has been used since as early as the 1950s by dentists in jaw reconstruction. Since the 1990s, it has also been widely used in plastic and orthopedic surgery as well as in dentistry for wound healing. According to Paul Christo, MD, in his book *Aches and Gains: A Comprehensive Guide to Overcoming Your Pain*,[2] The International Olympic Committee has suggested that PRP may be a serviceable option for treating athletic sports injuries, but it recommends proceeding with caution as more research is needed. To reiterate and add to what I listed earlier, current scientific evidence suggests the benefits of PRP use in patients with tennis elbow, plantar fasciitis, rotator cuff tendinitis, jumper's knee (patellar tendinitis), and other tendinopathies. In my opinion, if it's good enough for Olympic athletes, then it's good enough for people with an average activity level.

Augmenting the Golden Triad for Pain Relief

When the expected results are not achieved with The Golden Triad for Pain Relief, I will then use PRP. It's not the first choice of injection I routinely offer, mostly because it is not only more expensive than neural trigger point therapy, oxygen-ozone therapy, or PEMF therapy, but also because The Golden Triad for Pain Relief is so efficient that I don't usually need it.

There are no reported side effects with PRP because it comes from the patient's own blood. One reason why I may be getting superior results compared with what is reported in some studies is because I activate the PRP with oxygen-ozone. This serves to help release the growth factors and cytokines from the platelets so they can go where they are needed to reduce inflammation and promote tissue healing. The ozone also helps release the antioxidants from the PRP cells.

We recommend patients follow special procedures before the blood draw. These include a vegetarian diet at least twenty-four to forty-eight hours prior. This diet avoids the high cholesterol found in the PRP after a high-fat meal of red meat, for instance. Avoidance of foods that thin the blood (for example, ginger, garlic, and ginseng) is also highly recommended. The patient needs to come prepared by fasting for at least two hours. This also reduces the amount of cholesterol in the blood. If you take a daily aspirin, we ask you to check with your doctor to see if you can suspend this intake for two days prior to treatment. Steroids and NSAIDs (non-steroidal anti-inflammatory drugs like Motrin® or Advil®) can interfere with PRP's effects, so they are not recommended before or after the injection.

Oxygen-ozone mixed with PRP is a rule of thumb when I inject with PRP. I also use calcium chloride, which helps to do the same as ozone: it aids the release of growth factors and cytokines to go to work immediately and help repair and relieve pain. The results can be superior when compared with ozone as used by itself. PRP stimulates the growth of collagen, which is a main component of connective tissue like tendons and cartilage.

According to Dr. Nathan Wei in his book *The Book On PRP*, "PRP does not provide the instant pain relief that a cortisone injection might. However, unlike cortisone, PRP leads to healing of previously unhealthy tissue."[3] For this reason, I prefer it to cortisone injections.

I use the PRP not only to inject joints, but also for injecting soft tissue much the same way as the neural trigger point therapy. However, if the injecting doctor is not trained in neural trigger point therapy, then she will not be able to help you with localized trigger point injections using PRP.

Regenerative Medicine

Mesenchymal stem cell

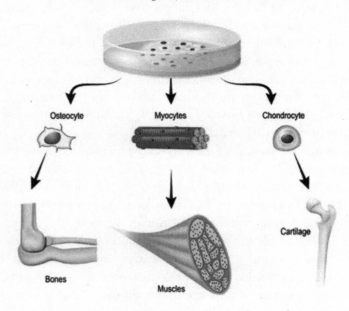

Mesenchymal stem cells (MSCs) are gaining popularity in regenerative medicine, and the term has entered the popular lexicon. Three types of MSCs are reported in the literature: bone marrow–derived (BM-MSCs), adipose-derived (AD-MSCs), and umbilical cord–derived (UC-MSCs). When administered to a tissue that is damaged, MSCs are multipotent, meaning that they can turn into a variety of cell types, including bone cells, cartilage cells, muscle cells, and fat cells.

The least invasive type of MSCs that a primary care doctor can use are umbilical cord–derived MSCs. These come from the umbilical cord of a healthy baby born in the United States and from consenting parents. The MSCs are harvested and processed by an FDA-registered lab; FDA-registered labs follow the same steps and procedures as that of organ transplant labs; as a result, the MSCs are screened for all kinds of infections.

The main advantage of UC-MSCs is that there is no blood type matching required between the stem cells and the patient receiving them. The other benefit is that there is no surgical procedure involved to harvest them as there is with bone marrow–derived or adipose-derived MSCs. In other words, the patient is not subjected to an additional surgical method of collecting the MSCs from the bone marrow or the patient's fatty tissues.

PRP and UC-MSC Treatments

The first reported successful use of UC-MSCs was in the case of a six-year-old boy with Fanconi's syndrome (i.e., inadequate reabsorption in tubules of the kidneys) in the late 1980s. The literature shows promising results in the regeneration of cartilage and disc tissue in osteoarthritis and lumbar disc disease. In my office, I use it for joint repair in the knees, hips, shoulders, and ankles. I even use it in cases of musculoskeletal and tendinitis conditions. The patient in question usually has not been responsive to The Golden Triad for Pain Relief and PRP. Therefore, I use this as a last resort as it is the most expensive of treatments. That said, the results can be outstanding, especially in the case of osteoarthritis and cartilage damage. Again, when you compare the expense of this treatment to joint replacement surgery, it's a very worthwhile, cost-effective investment in your health.

When I perform UC-MSC injections on patients, I invariably will use oxygen-ozonated PRP first to help the stem cells stay in the spot I'm injecting. In that way, they can go to work helping to regenerate the damaged or inflamed tissue. Perhaps that is why I see superior results when I use UC-MSCs given that I utilize oxygen-ozone and PRP with the procedure. Dr. Nathan Wei in his PRP book says: "To use an analogy, PRP—particularly when used in conjunction with stem cells—sends the healing process into 'warp drive.'"[4] Together with oxygen-ozone, I believe the healing process is definitely accelerated.

Contraindications to PRP injections include the following: blood and bleeding disorders, chronic liver disease, sepsis (infection of the blood), acute and chronic infections, blood thinner therapy (if you cannot go off it for the treatment), anemia, and pregnancy.

Relative contraindications to PRP are as follows: smokers, diabetics, those with compromised microcirculation, and anyone on immunosuppressive therapy.

PRP and UC-MSC injections are gaining popularity for treating many pain conditions. The emerging research into these two treatments is showing promise. Again, a pain patient should first try any of The Golden Triad for Pain Relief procedures, like PEMF, neural trigger point therapy, and oxygen-ozone therapy. Only if they have limited or no success with these, then they should be offered the PRP and, if need be, UC-MSCs. There are some dietary steps you can follow to increase your chances of success should you go for PRP alone or UC-MSCs. A patient who comes to me asking for stem cell injection will get PRP and oxygen-ozone at the same time to further enhance a positive outcome. As stated in the disclaimer to this book, MSCs have not been approved by the FDA, and therefore, we don't make any claims as to their ability to cure any condition.

CHAPTER 8

The Granddaddy of Them All: Headaches

"My migraines laugh at Advil."
—www.thedailymigraine.com

Headaches are among the most common forms of chronic pain and nervous system disorders. According to the World Health Organization (WHO), 50 to 75 percent of the world's adult population ages eighteen to sixty-five experienced a headache during the last year, and of those, at least as many as 30 percent reported migraines. Up to 4 percent have a headache fifteen days per month. Headaches affect all ages, races, incomes, and localities.[1] In the 2016 Global Burden of Disease Study (GBD), it was confirmed "that headache, and in particular, migraine, is a large public health problem in both sexes and all age groups worldwide."[2]

Recurrent headache disorder is associated with a considerable burden of personal and societal pain, disability, and loss of quality of life. Of course, the dire financial cost should go without saying. Some of the most common types of headache disorders include migraine headache and tension-type headache (TTH).

Migraines

Migraines begin at puberty for some, but they mostly affect those between the ages of thirty-five to forty-five years of age. There is a two-to-one prevalence ratio between women and men for this type of headache. So, one might suspect a hormonal component at the root of this troubling equation.[3]

The attacks are typically recurrent. For some women, their menstrual cycle is the trigger for the migraine. The attack is usually preceded by an aura, which is a sensory experience that besets an individual with light flashes or changes in vision. Often, it is a one-sided headache that is throbbing or pulsatile. Nausea is another common symptom. A migraine can last a few hours to several days. For some people, it literally stops them in their tracks—everything that they are doing comes to a grinding halt. The only recourse for sufferers is to find a place to lie down where it's very quiet and dark.

Tension-Type Headache (TTH)

TTH is the most common headache disorder. This variation can last a few hours up to several days. If it occurs on fewer than fifteen days a month, then it is considered episodic. If it occurs on greater than fifteen days a month, then it is considered chronic. TTH begins in the teens, and for every three women, two men suffer. Again, a hormonal component is suspected as a root cause. Stress and neck strain are also possible etiological factors. Chronic TTH can be unremitting and more disabling. It causes an individual to feel pressure or the sensation of a tight band around the head, and it can spread from the back of the neck to the brow.

Yvonne's Story: Headaches with Anxiety

"I first started experiencing severe chronic headaches five years ago. I was thirty years old at the time. I had headaches before this, but they were random and tolerable. These headaches now were different and more painful. I would be in tears, and often I would throw up. I tried several over-the-counter medications: Advil®, Tylenol®, Motrin®, Excedrin®, etc. These did not help my pain, and instead, my stomach became sensitive from all these different medications. I ended up in the emergency room (ER) on several occasions, without any help. The ER physician usually gave me a shot of a medicine that did not work. My primary care doctor referred me to a neurologist.

"The neurologist ordered the MRI and prescribed me muscle relaxants. I think it is important to note that I suffer from anxiety, and I am not a fan of medications, especially the ones that make me feel in any way 'off,' as this will trigger an anxiety attack. The muscle relaxant took the edge off, so I was no longer in tears or dizzy from the headache, but I was very sleepy and still felt the headache lingering. I did not like this side effect, so I decided to hold off on taking that medication further until the results of the MRI came back.

"At my follow-up appointment, I was told that I had a sinus problem that was causing my headaches. I was not surprised. I was prescribed more muscle relaxants and a nasal spray to use daily. I turned down both as I already had a prescription nasal spray from my primary care doctor for allergies/sinuses. The neurologist then offered me another medication to try, but after researching its side effects, I decided against it too.

"So, I kept going to the ER for my headaches, where I was sent home with medications that made my stomach upset, and I was nauseated with lightheadedness as well. On a scale of one to ten, my headaches were a nine or ten out of ten, and they were now lasting daily from a few hours to a few days. I was no longer living a normal life as the pain was so debilitating, and the smallest thing could trigger a headache. It was affecting every part of my life, and I felt depressed.

"A friend of mine whose chronic pain was fully resolved with Dr. Hirani's help referred me to her. I first saw Dr. Hirani in 2017. She is warm and understanding and takes her patients' pain symptoms seriously. I say this because she was not going to let me leave her office until I was completely pain free.

"She gave me two pain treatments that day: the abdominal injection and the intravenous procaine. The abdominal injection took away my anxiety immediately. I felt calm and relaxed. The IV procaine took away my headache completely within seconds. I was in shock and stayed in her office for a little while after these treatments as Dr. Hirani wanted to make sure the headache did not return.

"I can say that finding Dr. Hirani and her treatments have given me my life back. I can function normally without being in constant pain. I now return monthly for an abdominal injection to treat the anxiety and about every two to three months for the IV procaine when I feel a headache coming on. Both these treatments have helped my headaches and anxiety in ways I can't even explain to you. I was unable to leave my house most days, let alone walk into a store or restaurant prior to these treatments. Now, I can do this and so much more. I will continue going for these treatments as needed and will forever be grateful for her and the neural trigger point therapy."

Headache Treatments

The accepted method of treatment includes medications, lifestyle modifications (for example, stress reduction and smoking cessation), and patient education. If a patient is experiencing a headache while in my office, she will immediately get a B12 with magnesium intramuscular shot in the hip, which will quite often abort the headache. If necessary, then a procaine IV push will be administered.

The role of magnesium in neurological diseases has been known and studied for three decades. Magnesium is involved in nerve transmission and neuromuscular conduction. It is a mineral of interest in neurological disorders. A 2018 article in the journal *Nutrients* titled "The Role of Magnesium in Neurological Disorders" cited the following: "There is strong data to suggest a role for magnesium in migraine and depression, and emerging data to suggest a protective role for magnesium for chronic pain, anxiety, and stroke . . . Overall, the mechanistic attributes of magnesium in neurological diseases connote the micromineral as a potential target for neurological disease prevention and treatment."[4]

According to a set of United States guidelines in 2012 for prevention of migraines, magnesium was classified as level B.[5] Vitamin B12 levels have been shown in one study to be low in children with TTH.[6] Its role in headache prevention and treatment is under investigation. Vitamin B12 and magnesium are very safe nutrients, and even if you cannot get them in an injectable form, you should be supplementing with them for headaches. There are other vitamins and nutrients that have been studied for headache disorders, but that is not the focus of this particular book.

If the B12/magnesium injection is not successful in relieving the headache, then an IV procaine push (rapid, one-time intravenous administration) may do the trick. I have said this earlier—I am all about bringing instant pain relief to the patient. If the above two methods fail, then the patient will get a PEMF treatment; in this case, the coils are placed on the head, back of the neck, or on the particular area of the head where the pain is being experienced.

If that fails to bring about resolution, then the neural trigger point therapy bleb injections will be applied to the trigger points (tender spots) around the back of the neck (which is a source of most chronic tension-type headaches). In general, headache patients will usually leave our office with either partial or complete relief.

If the neural trigger point therapy blebs are not successful at bringing about significant improvement in the headache, then, of course, I will call in my "King of pain relief"—oxygen-ozone. The oxygen-ozone injections will follow in the same area of the procaine blebs. They are usually tiny injections. If you recall, one of ozone's mechanisms of action is to shut off the pain receptors at the cellular level, relieving the pain.

All patients suffering from headaches—whether of the migraine or tension type—are prescribed the elimination diet. I recall one patient returning for a follow-up visit in tears of joy and telling me that by eliminating gluten from her diet, she no longer had headaches. I've had patients tell me that by doing the elimination diet, they discovered that sugar triggers the migraine.

So, if you are a headache patient, you owe it to yourself to try to initially eliminate dairy, sugar, and gluten—or at the very least just wheat. These are the three most inflammatory foods I mentioned earlier. If after three weeks of completely avoiding these foods you are still experiencing headaches, then I would recommend trying the complete elimination diet referenced in the third chapter of this book.

Food Allergies, Sensitivities, and Nutritional Deficiencies

A blood test for food allergies (IgE) and food sensitivities (IgG) is done for the headache patient who I suspect may have allergies or sensitivities. If I suspect the headache is due to hormonal imbalances, then I will run a hormone panel (blood test) for a menstruating female on day twenty-one of the cycle, which is when the hormone progesterone peaks. If I find the progesterone level in the blood is low, then a trial of bioidentical progesterone cream is prescribed to the female patient. This is applied topically on the skin around the second half of her cycle, close to the onset of the headaches.

I will also check for nutritional deficiencies of magnesium and vitamin B12. Correcting nutritional deficiencies can also help a great deal for my headache patients. Stress reduction is of primary importance, but many of my patients seem oblivious to it or don't recognize how important a factor it is in one's health.[7] It is apparent to me that patients want to find an external cause for their pain and refuse to look internally to see if there is any psychological or emotional imbalance that is playing an additional role.

If the patient had success with neural trigger point therapy injections (with or without oxygen-ozone injections) or the IV push of procaine, they are strongly encouraged to return and do a full neural trigger point therapy session. This session can very often bring about a profound reduction in anxiety, which then leads to a reduction in headaches (I just spoke about stress playing a role in chronic pain, remember?).

A full neural trigger point therapy session almost always includes the IV procaine push. The abdominal injection (an intramuscular injection near the belly button area) is included in the full session and addresses the adrenal glands. The adrenals produce the hormone responsible for the fight-or-flight response that can lead to stress and anxiety. Sometimes, these two injections are all a patient needs for headaches. We know that there is a probable hormonal component in women. So, the pelvic injection in the groin region (see Chapter 12 on pelvic pain and its accompanying photo of procedure) not only helps with premenstrual syndrome (PMS), but it may also help reduce or eliminate headaches associated with it.

Sinus congestion as a cause of headaches is not reported much in the literature, but I see it often. Excedrin® manufacturers also know it's a common problem, which is the reason behind their sinus formulation. When a patient complains about pain along the forehead or the face, I examine the patient. If I find tenderness over the sinuses (like the frontal and maxillary sinuses), then I suspect this is a sinus headache patient.

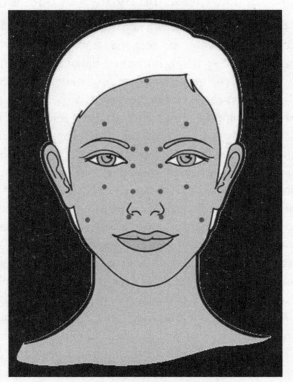

Example of the sinus pattern for neural trigger point blebs.

This particular type of patient must be willing to explore possible food intolerances (also known as food sensitivities) or allergies and try the anti-inflammatory diet. If the patient needs imaging to rule out chronic sinusitis, then I will refer them for imaging. PEMF therapy is administered first, and if the pain persists, then the sinus pattern (see diagram on previous page) with procaine is administered. If necessary, it will be followed by oxygen-ozone injections along the sixteen acupuncture points for sinus disorders.

PRP and UC-MSCs would be the next prescriptions for the chronic headache patient if the above treatments and recommendations were unsuccessful. These two treatments are definite game changers as well as cost-effective in the long term.

CHAPTER 9

Get Back in Circulation: Chronic Low Back Pain (LBP)

"Pain is inevitable. Suffering is optional."

—Buddhist proverb

Chronic back pain is second to headaches as the most common chronic pain disorder. Sixty-five million Americans report recent episodes of back pain. Sixteen million adults in the United States experience persistent or chronic back pain.[1] As a result, many of these people are unable to function normally. The definition of chronic back pain is pain that persists for twelve weeks or more despite the treatment of the initial acute episode. Of those people with acute (new onset) LBP, 20 percent will develop chronic LBP within a year. It is the most common cause of job-related disabilities and a leading contributor to missed workdays. Unlike headache disorders, this condition affects men and women equally.

The pain can range from dull or constant to a sudden, sharp stabbing that can be incapacitating. It can begin abruptly due to an accident or lifting something heavy, or over time, can appear due to age-related changes of the spine. Risk factors for LBP include anxiety, depression (or stress), being sedentary, older age, weight gain, genetics (like ankylosing spondylitis), and occupation-related factors. The most common types of chronic back pain that I see in my office are non-specific muscular strain, muscular spasm, osteoarthritis, disc disease, and sciatica.

Treating Chronic LBP

Accepted treatments are hot and cold packs, especially for acute pain. Minimal bed rest is recommended, and it is better to continue with your regular exercises. Strength training, physical therapy, and various prescription anti-inflammatory as well as narcotic medications are recommended.

In my office, the anti-inflammatory diet and supplementation are the first prescription for patients with chronic back pain. The next thing for them is to try the non-invasive PEMF therapy, which can be very effective for acute forms of back pain.[2] Sometimes it works for chronic back pain as well. The next step, according to The Golden Triad for Pain Relief, is the minimally invasive neural trigger point therapy (if the PEMF therapy was ineffective).

Depending on the patient's history, imaging studies, and physical exam, I will perform injections accordingly. After doing a thorough exam of my patient's back, which involves looking at the range of motion of the back, deformities, swelling, redness, and motor strength as well as palpating for muscular pain, I will perform the neural trigger point therapy.

For example, if it appears that the patient has just muscular strain, then the injections I deliver are of the superficial intradermal type (or blebs). This is done with a tiny needle and small amount of procaine at the trigger points. A discussion about tattoos, especially if you have one on your lower back where you have chronic back pain, is in order at this point.

Guess what? That tattoo is actually an interference field (discussed in Chapter 5 pertaining to neural trigger point therapy), and no matter how large or small, it needs the superficial procaine blebs of neural trigger point therapy. Scars from previous traumatic injuries or surgeries in the same area are also possible interference fields and require treatment in the same manner.

Paraspinal injections (intramuscular injections along either side of the spine) with procaine can be fantastic for chronic back pain if it is indicated by exam or imaging. It can help the muscular strain, osteoarthritis, disc disease, and radiculopathy patient.[3]

Procaine Injection Treatment

Just to recap, the anesthetic procaine will bring about temporary anesthesia or pain relief, but procaine breaks down quickly, and the anesthesia wears off quickly. If the patient is still pain free an hour after the treatment, you can be sure it is due to the neural trigger point therapy injection and not the effects of anesthesia. I tell the patient when leaving my office, "If you had twenty-four hours or more of pain relief before the pain returned, then that means this was a good treatment for you. The more sessions of treatment you do, the longer the duration of pain relief you will have."

As discussed previously, a patient will need an average of four to six sessions for full benefits. The patient may return as early as the following week for the second session. At this time, I will offer to use my "King of pain relief"—oxygen-ozone therapy. I first inject with procaine, then follow in the same area with the oxygen-ozone gas injection. If the patient had no results with just the neural trigger point therapy on the first visit (or the benefits were short-lived), then there is a high chance the patient will have a positive response to the oxygen-ozone injections.[4]

A Dentist's Story from Dr. C. D.: Chronic LBP

"I first met Dr. Hirani two years ago and discovered soon afterwards that she exemplifies what a physician ought to be. To begin with, she is very knowledgeable. She is always educating me on the latest developments in her field. She is generous in sharing her knowledge and often speaks at various medical seminars. That instilled a lot of confidence in me.

"Next, she took the time to listen to me. I have never felt rushed whenever I've come to an appointment. And I know she has a very busy practice. As a true holistic practitioner in the Los Angeles area, she is in high demand. Last but not least, she has a gentle touch, which is critical, especially when it comes to a needle-phobic patient.

"When I first came to Dr. Hirani, I had been dealing with low back pain for approximately fifteen years. Being a dentist only added to this particular matter. Long hours either hunched over in a chair or standing in one position was my usual day at the office. My back would go into a spasm, and I would be bedridden for the first few days, then remain out of alignment for a few weeks. Toward the end, it was happening with increased frequency. I would recover, only to have my back go out a couple of months later.

"Over the years, I had gone to the orthopedist twice, and a CT scan revealed a bulge in my disc, but no compression in my spine. Surgery was an option, but that didn't sound inviting to me. I shared my concern with Dr. Hirani, and she recommended an alternative approach.

"I was given the PEMF first, which is mild electrical stimulation to improve circulation. That was followed by oxygen-ozone injections along either side of my spine (intramuscular). I was doing physical therapy during this time as well. The PT, which I had been doing alone for many years, only provided me with short-term results. After only two treatments from Dr. Hirani, my back felt as good as new. Since then, I am happy to report that my back has not gone out. That was seven months ago. I can't thank her enough for the life-changing treatment she provided for me."

Iliopsoas Bursitis

Iliopsoas bursitis is a common chronic back and hip pain disorder I encounter, but there is little mention of it in medical literature. It is often underdiagnosed due to its unspecific symptomatology. The iliopsoas bursa sits over the front of the hip joint capsule. In about 14 percent of the population, it communicates with the hip joint. For this reason, it is often seen in association with conditions that cause chronic inflammation such as rheumatoid arthritis and osteoarthritis.

The iliopsoas is a muscle complex that makes up the hip flexor muscles of the body. Definitive diagnosis is made via imaging such as CT scan or MRI, which will show when the bursa is enlarged with fluid due to inflammation. Traditional therapies include non-steroidal anti-inflammatory medications, stretching exercises, steroid injections, aspiration (removal of the fluid in the bursa), and surgery if all else fails.

The psoas muscle attaches along the L1-L5 lumbar vertebrae and down to a section of the femur bone, so it is important to perform the paraspinal muscle injections over the area of L1-L5. First, I try with procaine; if that yields unsatisfactory results, then I will include the oxygen-ozone injection, which will usually yield the desired result.

Jen's Story: Iliopsoas Bursitis

"I began my journey with back and hip pain after a traumatic incident several years ago. Up until that time, I had led a very active lifestyle. Biking, hiking, skiing, and scuba diving were all activities that I enjoyed. This pain was unrelenting, and my physical movement became very limited. My left leg was weak and so stiff that I had to walk slowly because I couldn't put my left leg out in front of me very far. In the past, it was hard for people to keep up with me, but now people had to walk slowly so that I wasn't left behind, which made me feel very self-conscious and old.

"The pain was so bad initially that I was on steroids, muscle relaxers, and pain medication. My range of motion was very restricted, and I was limited in what I could do because of the pain. Carrying a bag of groceries hurt my hip. It made me see myself as helpless. Things I never needed help to do I now had to ask someone to do for me.

"As a nurse, I have a good understanding of pain, different types of pain, how it travels through the brain, and options for getting rid of it or living with it. I also know that if pain doesn't get better relatively quickly, then it becomes chronic and can last a lifetime. Mine had become chronic; it had been several years of pain along with physical limitations. I had epidurals, steroid trigger point injections, dry needling, pain medications, topical medications, physical therapy, hydrotherapy, acupuncture, a TENS unit, massage therapy, yoga, and even psychotherapy to see if it was all in my head.

"They all helped a little, but both the pain and lack of range of motion limited my life, changed my perception of myself, and made me sad with longing for getting my old life back. I was truly willing to do or try anything. What I have learned is that when you're ready, the Universe will bring you what you need if you listen.

"The Universe brought me Dr. Hirani. I had never heard of neural trigger point therapy; it did not make sense to me how procaine would help long term. I understood it as a numbing agent, but I wondered how something that numbs you for an hour was going to help my chronic pain and range of motion. She said, 'Just wait and see,' and she was very sure of herself.

"I laid down on the table with my butt facing the ceiling and she had me lift my legs one at a time. The left one barely came off the table, and the right one (unbeknownst to me) just raised up a little higher than my left. I didn't have any pain in that leg or hip, but because my range of motion was so diminished on my left, my right leg was indirectly affected. She started putting pressure on different areas of my lower back, butt, and legs, and almost every area was painful to pressure. Again, I had not realized that while my pain was being felt in one area, my whole lower back, butt, and thighs had been collateral damage.

"She proceeded to start injecting all the areas that were painful to touch with procaine and oxygen-ozone. She then had me raise my legs up off the table again, and I am not kidding when I say they both lifted up three times higher. I just started laughing and shaking my head! 'There is no way this is possible; nothing can do this!' It was like a magic trick, but I was the patient/assistant, so I knew it wasn't a trick. But I still just couldn't believe it! It was magic. Now I understood why she had said, 'Just wait and see.'

"It seemed to keep working after the injections because two weeks later I was even better. It did take numerous treatments, and I think it's important to understand that going into it if your pain is chronic. It took a long time for my body to get worse and deconditioned, and I had to commit to getting better and healthier. Rome was not built in a day, and while I got better in a day, it took months to gain the full advantage of what the neural trigger point therapy and oxygen-ozone could do to heal my body.

"I am back to being able to do the activities that I had enjoyed in the past. Do I still get some pain when I do too much? Sure, but there is no comparison to what I had experienced in the past. It's unfortunate that this therapy isn't mainstream medicine and that only very few people get to have it because it's not talked about a lot in medical journals. Neural trigger point therapy and oxygen-ozone by Dr. Hirani did not just help my pain, it allowed me to be me again. What's the value of that? Ask my family because they all LOVE Dr. Hirani for giving the real me back to them."

Sciatica

Sciatica is another debilitating form of chronic back pain that I see quite frequently. Sciatica is a pain that radiates down the back of the leg, starting in the lower back (lumbar spine) or sacral spine area. The accepted method of treatment is anticonvulsant and or anti-depressant medications. When these medications fail, then an invasive epidural injection is offered.

The patients I see with sciatica have not had success with these treatments. Remember that standard treatments for chronic pain have dismal results. We first offer sciatica patients the PEMF treatment as well as prescribed diet and supplements. Then comes the neural trigger point therapy. This is followed by the oxygen-ozone therapy if need be.

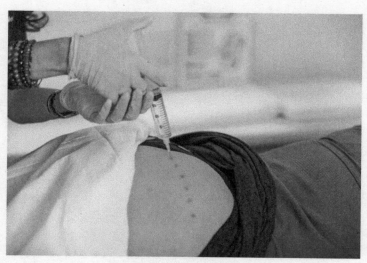

Neural trigger point blebs for sciatica.

This treatment for sciatica can be laborious. It requires that I painstakingly press along the path of the pain (trigger points) and superficially inject every tender spot with the procaine blebs (or saline if the patient does not want procaine).[5] A patient with sickle cell anemia has returned for this treatment several times. Overall, she has noticed that the degree of pain she now has is significantly diminished. To get faster results, I have also used oxygen-ozone on her.[6]

She has recently realized that dietary infractions and stress both trigger her pain—this should be especially noted by all nonbelievers in a diet/stress and pain connection. Finally, the number of injections she requires each time she comes has lessened. It is not surprising that she has better results when I combine neural trigger point therapy with oxygen-ozone. Remember, the injections performed on her are minimally invasive—almost like acupuncture. The time it takes to perform all the injections is significant (an hour sometimes), but the results are fantastic. The first time I did it for her, she went home and cried because she couldn't ever remember being free of pain, given that she had suffered from sciatica her entire life!

As with headache disorders, if The Golden Triad for Pain Relief was not successful enough or if the patient wants faster results and can afford PRP[7] or UC-MSCs,[8] then I will provide those. The results speak for themselves.

CHAPTER 10

Bone of Contention: Chronic Joint Pain

"When you get to the end of your rope,
tie a knot and hang on."

—Theodore Roosevelt

According to a 2017 article in the *British Medical Journal*, neck pain is in the top five of chronic pain disorders in terms of prevalence and years lost to disability.[1] The good news is that most acute episodes of neck pain resolve spontaneously. But more than a third of affected people still have low-grade symptoms or recurrences more than a year later. When the pain has lasted for more than twelve weeks, it's called chronic neck pain.

Different types of neck pain exist: the muscular type associated with sore muscles, muscle spasm where the patient experiences severe tightness, the headache type (see Chapter 8), and joint pain of the vertebrae in the cervical (neck) spine. If arthritis is causing the joint pain, then it is worse typically in the morning. This is a nerve pain type where the nerve roots from the cervical spine are compressed (or pinched) as they emerge from the spinal canal. Bone spurs from arthritis can cause this as well. Additionally, a herniated disc in the neck can cause nerve pain.

Neck Pain Treatments

Typical treatments are similar to those for back pain and include heat and ice, pain medications, physical therapy, and steroid injections. Surgery can also be offered; this depends on the type of neck pain and if other treatments have failed. In my office, we first offer PEMF therapy[2] along with the anti-inflammatory diet and supplements. In many cases, that is all that is needed.

If that initial approach doesn't work, then it's neural trigger point therapy time. I first check for interference fields (for example, scars or tattoos in the neck region). If there is pain upon pressing over the trapezius muscles, it's a sign that the tonsils are involved, and the patient gets a tonsillar injection (see Chapter 5). If addressing the interference fields was not enough with the patient still in pain, then I will do neural trigger point injections (where I find the tender spots on the patient's neck and inject each with a small needle and small amount of procaine [the blebs] as illustrated in photo in Chapter 5).

If the pain persists, then I will use oxygen-ozone injections next. On examination of the neck, if there is a spinal motor weakness to any or all of the C5, C6, or C7 (cervical spinal) nerves, then an intramuscular injection is performed in this area with procaine and oxygen-ozone. This injection requires specialized training. The injection is extremely helpful for the patient with neck joint pain like arthritis or nerve pain. Any adequately trained primary care doctor can perform these injections. The oxygen-ozone goes in and shuts off the pain receptors while stimulating the production of antioxidants to quell the inflammation.

Delivering successful injections to the neck requires knowledge of neural trigger point therapy as well as interference fields and how to eliminate them. The practitioner should know how to perform a comprehensive neck exam. The treatments are tiered, beginning with the least invasive (diet/supplements and PEMF therapy) and, if need be, proceeding to the minimally invasive neural trigger point therapy and/or oxygen-ozone. Finally, there are the PRP and UC-MSC therapies. These are used in cases where the results with PEMF therapy, neural trigger point therapy, and oxygen-ozone therapy are not as effective, or the patient wants faster relief.

Shoulder Pain Treatments

Shoulder pain is common, and many shoulder pain sufferers experience accompanying disability. A 2011 article in the journal *BMC Musculoskeletal*

Disorders reported an annual incidence of shoulder pain in primary care at 14.7 per 1,000 patients, with a lifetime prevalence of up to 70 percent. The article noted high recurrence rates, with 25 percent of shoulder pain sufferers reporting previous episodes, and 40 to 50 percent reporting persisting pain or recurrence at their twelve-month follow-up.[3]

Traditional treatment for chronic shoulder pain includes typical recommendations like pain medications, physical therapy, and steroid injections. However, activity modification is also a recommendation in cases of rotator cuff tendinitis. This includes no overhead activity, bench pressing, kayaking, or overhead throwing. Treatments at my office are the standard PEMF therapy[4] and anti-inflammatory diet/supplements.

In general, I find that these first two will provide some relief, but not 100 percent. Neural trigger point therapy is often required next. After performing a shoulder exam, I will palpate (or press over) common areas of tenderness and apply the procaine injection blebs there. If necessary, I will perform intra-articular injections (into the shoulder joint). Again, oxygen-ozone is employed if needed.[5]

The results with oxygen-ozone and procaine for shoulder pain are excellent. Patients may need several sessions depending on the severity. PRP[6] and UC-MSCs are used if The Golden Triad for Pain Relief didn't do the trick or the patient requested it.[7] The benefit of the injections mentioned above is that there is no restriction on how many treatment sessions you can have. When you get steroid (cortisone) injections, the limit is no more than three per year. That is not the case with neural trigger point therapy, oxygen-ozone, PRP, and UC-MSCs.

Patients can come every few weeks as needed until the pain is gone. Generally speaking, I tell patients to expect to have four to six sessions at a minimum. That said, every patient is unique, and the number of sessions needed will depend on the patient and what else she is doing to promote healing. When you have been suffering as long as you have without any answers, and you have finally found something that is working, you will understand the cost-efficient component of getting your life back.

Knee Pain Treatments

Based on National Health and Nutrition Examination Survey (NHANES) and Framingham Osteoarthritis Study (FOS) data,[8] the incidence of knee pain has increased. Osteoarthritis of the knee is the most common form of knee pain, and it is the most common form of osteoarthritis. Risk factors include being overweight, having sustained injury or infection (including repetitive stress injuries), age, and gender (women over age fifty-five are more likely than men to have it). The standard treatment is the usual application of heat/ice, pain medications, physical therapy exercises, and, if necessary, steroid injections to the knee.

My standard treatment is—you guessed it—PEMF therapy[9] and anti-inflammatory diet/supplements first. But there is something important you need to know about knee pain: Not all knee pain is due to osteoarthritis, and not all osteoarthritis of the knee is accompanied by pain. What this means is that if a patient comes to me with X-rays showing degeneration of the knee joint (as is seen in osteoarthritis), the pain may not be due to osteoarthritis. This fact is well known, but most doctors only see it as osteoarthritis and treat it as such. When conservative treatments, which include injections into the joint with steroids or hyaluronic acid, have failed, then the patient is sent for knee replacement surgery. I have seen plenty of patients with chronic knee pain that is not due to osteoarthritis at all, or their pain problem is related to something else.

If the patient is requiring neural trigger point therapy, I will palpate around the knee, looking for tender spots just like I have done for other chronic pain conditions. However, in the case where I find sore spots, sometimes I don't even need to inject with procaine blebs. I will inject these tiny blebs in the groin or inguinal region, and "miraculously" the pain on palpation around the knee is gone. You might think that I'm making this up. The only explanation is there may be a blocked lymphatic issue (since there are lymph nodes in the groin, which are connected to the nerve pathways). The knee pain can significantly improve after the treatment. (See the section on the lymphatics in Chapter 5).

The patient may even unknowingly have pain in the groin region that is only noticed upon palpation. If you are experiencing knee pain, try pressing around your groin area. If you experience pain there, the problem with your knee may not be arthritis—it may be a groin or lymphatic issue. *Believe it or not, looking for pain on palpation in the inguinal or groin region is part of the physical examination for the knee.* Sometimes, there is tenderness over the pes anserine bursa, which is an area medial to the knee and just above it. If I inject with procaine blebs, the pain can often disappear instantly.

Of course, if oxygen-ozone is needed, I will use it and most likely with phenomenal results. The bottom line is this: It is important to know that not all knee pain is due to osteoarthritis—even if your X-ray shows you have it. Many of my patients walk out of the office free of pain without even needing an intra-articular injection of oxygen-ozone[10] or procaine. PRP and UC-MSCs[11] are often used for intra-articular injection in cases of severe osteoarthritis of the knee with pain.[12] Research has shown benefits and may even prevent unnecessary knee joint replacement.

Rob's Story: Knee Pain

"I had a very active and physical life as a firefighter and athlete for over thirty years. The years of activity had caused a lot of damage to my left knee. I ended up having arthroscopic surgery on it with the hopes of easing some of the problems. Instead of things getting better, my knee got worse. I started having more pain throughout the day. The worst was the constant sharp pain when I tried to sleep. It didn't matter what I did at night, repositioning, or how many pillows I used. The severe, stabbing pain kept me up night after night.

"Trying to alleviate the pain, I got steroid injections into the knee and tried anti-inflammatory medications, but nothing seemed to ease the pain. My work was starting to be affected by the pain and lack of proper sleep. I was slower to get moving, tired, depressed, and started gaining weight, but most of all, I found my decision-making was affected. It was looking like I needed a knee replacement, and I felt like my career as a firefighter was coming to an end. I was considering retirement and spoke with my wife about it. She was not surprised as she'd seen the change in my attitude and how the pain was affecting me. I decided to go see Dr. Hirani as I had not tried anything alternative. She was highly recommended.

"I had to fly from Seattle to see her in Los Angeles. By this time, I had come to believe that nothing was going to help me. When Dr. Hirani saw me and examined me, she felt the problem was not with my knee joint, which was what all the other doctors thought it was. She believed it was a blockage in my lymphatic system. She recommended neural trigger point therapy and gave me a series of procaine injections to my groin area and around the knee. She also used oxygen-ozone injections. I didn't want to seem offensive, but I didn't see how this would help based on all the other treatments I had tried on the knee.

"The procedure took less than an hour, and afterward, I didn't feel any different. I went home thinking, 'Well, at least I gave it my best shot.' That night I found I still had the pain, but it seemed slightly less. It wasn't until the following night that I found I didn't have pain anymore! After nearly a year of dealing with this pain, it was suddenly gone.

"After a month, I noticed the pain started to come back again, but it was much less. I got on the plane and went back to see Dr. Hirani, and she treated me a second time, with procaine, oxygen-ozone, and PRP. Again, the pain was gone, this time for good, I hope. It's been a year, and I am still pain free. I am back to my active lifestyle, training at the gym, and my career as a firefighter. My physical and decision-making abilities are back. My physical limitation is no longer a factor in considering retirement. Knee surgery of course is not necessary anymore. I cannot express how thankful I am to Dr. Hirani with her care for my knee."

CHAPTER 11

When Nerves Attack:
Neuropathic Pain

"You just do it. You force yourself to get up. You force yourself
to put one foot before the other . . . you refuse to let it get you.
You fight. You cry. You curse. Then you go about your business
of living. That's how I've done it. There's no other way."

—Elizabeth Taylor

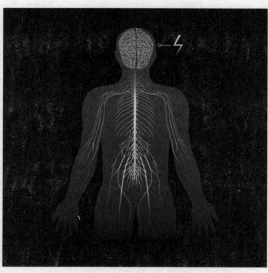

The path of nerves when they are inflamed.

Neuropathic pain is due to nerve damage or malfunctioning of the nervous system. It characteristically involves shooting pains, burning pain, tingling, and even numbness. The following medical conditions are associated with it: alcoholism, diabetes, amputation (phantom limb), chemotherapy, facial nerve disorders, AIDS (HIV), multiple myeloma, MS, shingles, and spine surgery. Treatments include antidepressant and anticonvulsant medications, NSAIDs (like ibuprofen), physical therapy, etc. It is widely known that patients have a poor response to standard treatments and, unfortunately, can get worse instead of better over time.

Fibromyalgia Treatments

Fibromyalgia is a widespread musculoskeletal pain that is dull and has lasted at least three months. It is accompanied by a variety of symptoms that include fatigue, brain fog (impaired memory and concentration), anxiety, depression, sleep disorders (restless leg syndrome or sleep apnea), TMJ, TTH, IBS, and bladder symptoms. Fibromyalgia does not originate as a muscle disease. Rather, it is a problem of central pain that comes from the central nervous system. Women are twice as likely to have it compared to men, and most people are diagnosed during middle age.[1]

Fibromyalgia patients make up 40 percent of all patients referred to our integrative medicine clinic. There is no evidence of a single trigger for fibromyalgia. It is usually associated with many possible triggers, which include the following: physical and emotional stressors, viral infection (patient will recall having a history of a preceding flu-like infection), and Lyme disease. Though suspect genes are still being explored, genetics also seem to play a role since the issue runs in families.[2]

Standard treatments for fibromyalgia include lifestyle adaptation of diet and exercise (data is especially supportive of the latter) and sleep management (this is key to breaking the cycle of pain). CBT, mindfulness classes and support groups, empathy (from the doctor), and pain management are other accepted forms of treatment. There is no convincing evidence for prescribing opioid pain medications in the management of fibromyalgia, yet so many patients are taking them.

Recommended medications are anti-depressants and anticonvulsants, which at the most can bring about 50 percent improvement in alleviating the pain. When I heard this at a pain management conference, I was both horrified and saddened because there are several effective, low-cost treatments that most doctors are unaware of. As a result, most patients will never get to experience the successful outcomes I've seen.

By now, you know what fibromyalgia patients are going to be prescribed by me—diet/supplements/PEMF therapy.[3] More than likely, they will also need neural trigger point therapy with oxygen-ozone[4] and potentially PRP or UC-MSCs.[5] These patients are some of the most complex I see in my practice, and they will need more than my standard go-to treatments. Their hormones are out of balance, so correcting this condition with bioidentical hormones is usually a necessary step.

Thyroid hormone replacement for these patients can be a game-changer. It can help with fatigue, depression, and pain. Anxiety and sleep must also be addressed. I recently received an email from a patient that said, "Neural trigger point therapy really helped my sleep, and I feel much calmer overall." This is a common response after neural trigger point therapy.

For some patients, when the pain level comes down, everything gets better. These patients have low cortisol[6] (I check this on all fibro patients). Treatment with adrenal support is beneficial. Testing for food allergies and sensitivities (IgE and IgG foods) is done if I suspect food plays a role. If positive, I will prescribe (and often with very good results) an elimination diet and a homeopathic or micro-dose-like treatment called low-dose allergen (LDA) therapy.

Low-Dose Naltrexone (LDN)

LDN is being studied in chronic pain disorders and showing promise.[7] LDN may be effective in reducing inflammation and blocking pain pathways. I often prescribe this medication, which has the added benefit of helping with sleep since it's a bedtime medication. LDN is a compounded medication and is not available at your regular pharmacy. A compounded medication is made from scratch and is not mass-produced like standard medications. A specialty compounding pharmacy will make it for you.

In its full strength, naltrexone is prescribed for drug or alcohol addiction. The low-dose formulation is a fraction of the original dose, similar to homeopathy or micro-dosing. LDN is thought to modulate the immune system and result in improvement of symptoms of fibromyalgia. There are few or no side effects with LDN. Ask your doctor for a prescription since there is science behind this recommendation.

Exercise is very important if you are a fibro patient. If you are limited in your ability to walk, then at least ask your doctor for a physical therapy prescription. Aquatic exercises can be helpful, too.

Sickle Cell Anemia

Of patients with sickle cell disease (SCD), 37 percent have neuropathic pain.[8] Sickle cell anemia is the most common inherited blood disorder in the United States.[9] A mutation in the hemoglobin molecule (which transports oxygen to the cells) causes the red blood cells to change their shape or become sickle-cell shaped.

These affected red blood cells can die early and cause anemia, but they can also block small blood vessels due to their abnormal shape. This can bring on a sickle cell crisis of severe pain. Patients with this crisis need to be in the hospital and get intravenous pain medications along with hydration. The latter helps to flush out the sickle cells.

Patients also need blood transfusions frequently. Sickle cell anemia patients are prone to infections, pain, and fatigue outside of their sickle cell crisis episodes. One out of five African Americans suffers from this disorder. Signs and symptoms begin in early childhood with repeated infections and pain. Standard treatments include pain medications like opioids and NSAIDs. Many who suffer from the condition have underlying pain all the time.

Rea's Story: Sickle Cell Crisis

My patient, Rea, who has SCD, had come to see me for chronic hip and sciatic pain. With The Golden Triad for Pain Relief approach, she had been getting better. However, she contacted me a while later to tell me that she was in the middle of a sickle cell crisis and wanted to avoid hospitalization. She wanted to know if I could help her, and I agreed to try. She came into my office three days in a row for IV saline hydration along with PEMF therapy, which took away her leg and back pain instantly. The IV saline ozone was another home run for her. Each time she came in, she felt so much better.

That particular week, she had to miss work. Still, by aborting the pain quickly and avoiding heavy narcotic IV pain medications and hospitalization, she rebounded to her usual self within a week. This was far more preferable to the standard two to three weeks of debilitation with hospitalization. It pains me that we could be relieving pain and restoring quality of life for those who suffer from SCD much more quickly. Additionally, we could be saving millions of dollars by avoiding hospitalization for sickle cell crisis. By just providing outpatient IV saline hydration and PEMF therapy— which now has so much scientific support—a lot of money could be saved.

Multiple Sclerosis (MS)

MS can be a very debilitating disease of the central nervous system (which involves the brain and spinal cord). In MS, the immune system attacks the myelin sheath that wraps around the nerves. This can result in misfiring and miscommunication of the neurons with the rest of the body. Nearly one million cases exist in the United States (and 2.3 million globally). Women are three times as likely to acquire it compared with men, and the average age of onset is between twenty and fifty years.[10,11]

Symptoms vary from none during the patient's lifetime to severe chronic symptoms or recurrent attacks of inflammation of the central nervous system. These symptoms include numbness and tingling, visual problems, spasticity of muscles, problems with walking, dizziness, vertigo, depression, anxiety, constipation, fatigue, bladder problems, weakness, sexual dysfunction, and pain. A 2007 study showed that up to 80 percent of MS patients experience neuropathic pain due to damage of the central nervous system.

Joy's Story: MS

"I was diagnosed with multiple sclerosis in 2017. Anyone with this disease will know that it affects everyone in different ways. For me, I have it in my neck, arms, and legs, where I initially suffered from such chronic pain that I was bedridden for six months. I was afraid of being reliant on pain medications, but I could not bear the heavy electrical pain, which was so bad that I could not even use my arms to wash my hair. I had difficulty brushing my teeth and flushing the toilet with my right arm due to heavy tendinosis.

"I started neural trigger point therapy, and to my utter amazement, after just four rounds of treatment along with PRP, I got full rotation back with my arms. I experienced such miraculous results that I was able to stop the tramadol (narcotic pain medication) and supplements for pain as well. I have continued neural trigger point therapy by itself on average every four to six weeks over the past two years and have gained more strength and mobility.

"Where pain used to be my biggest complaint, it is now the least of my complaints. My 'heavy legs' syndrome has improved, and I can use my legs for a longer period of time now. Neural trigger point therapy has been the single most effective MS treatment I have ever received. It has enabled me to stay off pain medications and allowed me to function on a daily basis. Prior to this treatment, I was virtually unable to do anything. I think it's the best kept secret when it comes to life-changing, alternative pain relief methods."

Complementary and Alternative MS Treatments

The exact cause of MS is unknown. Established risk factors include vitamin D deficiency, smoking, and obesity in childhood. Epstein-Barr virus is also emerging as a possible etiological agent. There is no cure. There are a lot of medications that are FDA approved to modify the course of the disease and treat the various symptoms. When it comes to pain management in MS, this includes steroids for relapses or attacks, muscle relaxants, anticonvulsants like Neurontin®, antidepressants, and antispasmodics. Physical therapy can also be helpful. Pain in MS affects sleep and activities of daily living. Quality of life is impacted greatly.

A 2018 study published in the journal *Neurología* found that PEMF therapy given to MS patients showed a significant improvement in their pain and quality of life.[12] Every MS patient suffering from pain deserves a trial of PEMF therapy. If PEMF therapy is not so effective, then neural trigger point therapy along with oxygen-ozone most likely will bring about significant pain relief.

A 2007 study published in the *Journal of Alternative and Complementary Medicine* looked at neural trigger point therapy in MS. They found that 65 percent of the MS patients in the pilot study and 76 percent of the MS patients in the double-blind, placebo-controlled, randomized study benefitted from the neural trigger point therapy. The locations of the tiny procaine blebs were around acupuncture points at the ankles and also at the largest circumference of the skull (crown of thorns pattern).[13] In my practice in treating MS, I usually administer more blebs than in just these two locations.

European studies have demonstrated increased cerebral blood flow in MS patients after IV oxygen-ozone therapy.[14,15] The thinking is that if blood flow and oxygen concentration are increased with IV oxygen-ozone therapy, then the pathophysiology or demyelination process may be improved, halted, or reversed. IV saline ozone therapy is discussed in Chapter 6, and has been shown to be safe and potentially quite therapeutic for inflammatory conditions.

Shingles or Postherpetic Neuralgia (PHN)

One million cases of PHN have been estimated to occur annually in the United States.[16] One in three will develop shingles in their lives.[17] PHN is a neuropathic pain syndrome that can last for months to years after the initial shingles or zoster rash. Shingles is a reactivation of the dormant chickenpox virus if you had it as a child. This reactivation is commonly found along a dermatome (or strip of nerves) that wraps around either side of your torso. It can also occur in other areas of the body. Blisters pop up and can be very painful. PHN is the most common complication of shingles. It affects the nerves and the skin, causing burning pain that lasts long after the shingles rash and blisters are gone.

PHN Treatments

Standard treatments include anticonvulsant medications, antidepressants, and opioid pain medications. PEMF therapy can be effective in treating this condition. In one study, neural trigger point therapy, combined with selected medications along with acupuncture and cupping therapy, resulted in a 75 to 100 percent improvement in pain from PHN.[18]

A 2018 study published in the *Journal of Pain Research*[19] compared a group of PHN patients treated alone with standard pharmacological (prescription medications) therapy and a group of PHN patients given the pharmacological therapy as well as IV oxygen-ozone therapy. The group of patients who received the combination pharmacologic and ozone had better outcomes. This article demonstrates that in some cases, if you combine the standard medical treatments with CAM treatments, the results can be superior. In other words, I am in full support of patients continuing with their standard pharmacological regimens while they are receiving CAM treatments in my office.

So, if you are suffering from PHN and have achieved some degree of improvement with your standard anticonvulsive medication, for example, it is not necessary for you to come off this medication in order to try oxygen-ozone therapy or neural trigger point therapy. These treatments are extremely safe, and they can easily be combined with standard pharmacotherapy. For my patients, I get positive results with my standard combination of neural blebs followed by oxygen-ozone injections to the painful trigger points for PHN. The IV saline ozone therapy is always recommended to patients suffering from chronic pain, and the results are always better than if they didn't do it.

Diabetes and Diabetic Peripheral Neuropathy (DPN)

Approximately 10 percent of the adult population in the United States suffers from diabetes.[20] Diabetic peripheral neuropathy (DPN) is the most common complication associated with diabetes. Approximately 50 percent of diabetic adults will be affected by DPN, which is the leading cause of disability due to foot ulceration, amputation, and difficulty walking, with increased risk of falls and injury. A 2016 study in *F1000Research* noted the annual cost of diabetes at over $245 billion, with 27 percent of this cost attributable to DPN.[21]

Symptoms of DPN include loss of pain sensation, tingling, the sensation of pins and needles, burning, and electric shock. Research shows that improvement of diabetes control, diet, exercise, and weight loss (if obese) can slow the progression of DPN. Foot care to prevent ulcers and physical therapy when necessary can also help.

DPN Treatments

Oxidative stress or inflammation is considered the underlying mechanism of DPN. Alpha-lipoic acid (a supplement) is considered the most successful antioxidant in clinical trials and is approved for treatment of DPN in Europe.[22] I prescribe this supplement to any patient with neuropathy. DPN is, for the most part, considered irreversible. Treatment is focused on blood sugar control, foot care, and pain management. The medications prescribed are the typical ones I have covered for other neuropathic pain conditions, namely anticonvulsants like Neurontin® and antidepressants.

PEMF therapy has been studied in DPN with successful outcomes. One study that was published in 2016 in the journal titled *Practical Pain Management* used PEMF therapy weekly on DPN patients for eight weeks consecutively and resulted in 52 percent improvement in pain and 65 percent improvement in sensory loss.[23] Every patient with DPN gets a PEMF trial at my office.

Since the peripheral (superficial) nerves are affected in DPN, neural trigger point therapy is worth trying on these patients along with oxygen-ozone therapy if necessary. Oxygen-ozone therapy is used frequently to treat diabetic foot ulcers, with very good results, and I have seen it heal a patient's foot ulcer firsthand. Many studies have been published showing the ability of oxygen-ozone therapy to heal the ulcers.

DPN is a state of oxidative stress. It makes sense that oxygen-ozone could help the DPN by increasing the availability of antioxidants in the body that reduce the oxidative stress or inflammation. Every patient who comes to my office is offered a trial of IV saline ozone in addition to oxygen-ozone injections.

CHAPTER 12

South of the Belly Button: Chronic Pelvic Pain (CPP)

"Being able to walk pain free is a blessing. Being able to walk without showing the pain is a skill."

—Kylie McPherson

Chronic pelvic pain in women is experienced in the area between the belly button and hips and lasts more than six months. This persistent pain is unrelated to the menstrual cycle. There are multiple causes for CPP including medical conditions unrelated to the pelvic region. Often, when these conditions are treated, the pain may resolve.

CPP is typically associated with other somatic pain syndromes such as irritable bowel and chronic fatigue syndromes as well as mental health conditions like post-traumatic stress disorder (PTSD) and depression. Diagnosis of CPP is made based on a patient's personal medical history and physical exam. A pelvic ultrasound can be done to evaluate for anatomical abnormalities, and in severe cases, the patient has to undergo a laparoscopic surgery to look for endometriosis.

Finding a cure for CPP is elusive and evidence-based therapies are limited to date. These include depot medroxyprogesterone, gabapentin, NSAIDS, gonadotropin-releasing hormone antagonists, pelvic floor PT, and behavioral therapy. In my experience, a hysterectomy remains a last resort.

Female Pelvic Pain

Chronic pelvic pain (CPP) affects one in seven women in the United States.[1] Pelvic pain is responsible for 10 percent of all referrals to the gynecologist.[2] Menstrual cramps, ovulation, GI issues (e.g., food intolerances), urinary issues, endometriosis, ovarian cysts, uterine fibroids, and disorders of the muscles and ligaments of the pelvic floor are some of the common reasons for CPP.

The associated pain lasts for more than six months and is linked to other syndromes like IBS, chronic fatigue syndrome, post-traumatic stress disorder, and depression. Doctors will perform an ultrasound to rule out any anatomical abnormalities. Then laparoscopy, a surgical procedure looking for endometriosis, is done next. When tissue from the uterus is located outside of the uterus and is causing severe pain, it is called endometriosis.

Delany's Story: Pelvic Pain

"My pelvic pain started when I was twelve and a half years old and started my period. I am now sixteen. The pain would start a day before my period and last throughout the entire duration of the period. The pain grade ranged from eight to ten out of ten at all times and was excruciating. It would leave me in tears all the time. I remember feeling very depressed and down just at the thought of having to deal with this pain for the rest of my life.

"At first, I didn't tell my mom how bad it was because I was afraid to go to the doctor. I would spend the entire time of my period in bed. After a few months, I finally told my mom, and she gave me a heating pad to try, but it didn't help. She then gave me Motrin®, which was also not helpful. Tylenol® was of no help either. At this point, my mom would send me to school regardless of how much pain I was in. She said, 'You cannot miss a week of school every month!' I would leave the house in tears on my way to school.

"My mom took me to the pediatrician, who recommended over-the-counter Midol® even though she knew we had tried Motrin® and Tylenol® already. So, I tried it, again with no pain relief. I remember calling my mom from school one day crying because the pain was unbearable, and the Midol® did nothing for me.

"At this point, I was feeling hopeless and depressed. My mom picked me up from school, and I know she was sad because she didn't know what else to do for me. I eventually started staying home from school during my periods and missed a lot of schoolwork. Now, I had even more stress from missed schoolwork. My pediatrician then gave me extra-strength ibuprofen.

She said this would help since it was stronger than the over-the-counter ibuprofen. It did help a little at first, but it did not take the pain away.

"My mom found Dr. Hirani, who uses neural trigger point therapy for pain relief. At first, I was skeptical since nothing had worked me thus far, and I refused to go. My mom did not give up and continued to ask me to see Dr. Hirani. I finally agreed and saw her for the first time this year. She did the pelvic injection and a few others. After the first session, my pain was completely gone within a few hours. The next month of my cycle, I waited for the pain to return, and it never did. Honestly, I was shocked because I felt like there was no hope for me. I will always be grateful for finding Dr. Hirani and her team. I feel so comfortable with her and am amazed at how she can help people suffering from life-changing pain. She helped end years of pain and suffering for me."

CPP Treatments

Treatment for CPP includes hormones, Neurontin®, NSAIDs, CBT, neuromodulation, and physical therapy offering pelvic floor exercises. Significant improvement occurs in only half of the cases. If the uterus is involved, then a hysterectomy is done only as a last resort. Iris Kerin Orbuch, MD, and Amy Stein, DPT, have written an excellent book titled, *Beating Endo: How to Reclaim Your Life from Endometriosis*.[3] It has a lot of practical suggestions for managing the pain. I am always interested in relieving pain in the quickest, safest way possible.

I conduct a thorough history and exam and order appropriate functional medicine tests, such as stool analysis and food allergy and sensitivity tests for women with GI- or IBS-type symptoms. If I suspect a hormonal component, then hormones are measured, too. Correcting hormonal imbalances can improve symptoms like vaginal dryness, which can lead to painful intercourse in some perimenopausal or menopausal women.

If the exam reveals abdominal (tummy) pain on palpation of the stomach, then neural trigger point therapy is offered first. Most of the injections are procaine blebs. Keep in mind that the patient is already on the anti-inflammatory diet/supplements and has already tried PEMF therapy. This latter treatment can also help with bladder symptoms.[4] If there is inguinal (groin) pain upon examination, then the procaine blebs are applied in that area.

An MD radiologist patient of mine experienced CPP following childbirth. She was told that the pubic symphysis (cartilaginous joint that holds the right and left pubic bones together) was separated, and as a result, nothing could be done and that she "just had to live with it." When I examined her, she had inguinal pain, and the procaine blebs I performed over this area instantly got rid of her pain, and it never came back. It turned out that the symphysis pubis dysfunction (SPD) was not the correct diagnosis. In truth, doctors are not taught to look for inguinal (groin) pain as a possible etiological cause of pain, nor are they shown that a simple technique of procaine blebs in the groin could eliminate the pain.

The pelvic (Frankenhauser plexus) injection is a significant injection for CPP patients, especially women.[5,6] It is a neural trigger point therapy injection that has done wonders for this kind of pain. Women will get up off the treatment table in total disbelief that their pain is gone. In addition, the pelvic injection will help either greatly diminish or completely eliminate those dreaded, monthly menstrual cramps and ovulation pain. Back and stomach pain will be greatly diminished or gone as well.

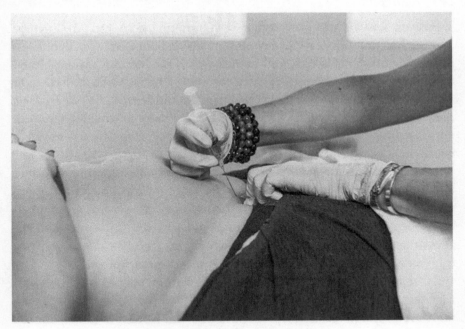

Example of pelvic injection.

For many women, the libido that had been waning or disappeared has suddenly come back! Hot flashes can be resolved or greatly diminished. Dyspareunia (pain with intercourse) can also get better from neural trigger point therapy. This treatment alone for CPP is so effective that I rarely need to utilize the oxygen-ozone injections except for women with abdominal pain associated with the CPP. Then, oxygen-ozone is my go-to "King of pain relief."

I remind the patient that she may need to return to have a few more sessions to reset the nerves in the pelvic area permanently. C-section scars can be a source of pain and must be treated with neural trigger point therapy (as discussed in Chapter 5 under scars). I had one patient with chronic perineal pain who never told me about her clitoral ring until I examined her. I recommended immediate removal of the ring and gentle procaine blebs over the area. She agreed to it, and needless to say, she got better.

Male Chronic Prostatitis/Chronic Pelvic Pain Syndrome (CP/CPPS)

According to a 2016 study, CP/CPPS in males makes up 90 percent of outpatient visits to the urologist,[7] and it is a complex and challenging condition to treat. There is no clearly established, effective treatment regimen. Worldwide, it has up to a 16 percent prevalence in men below fifty years of age.[8] Of course, they experience a poor quality of life. It goes without saying that all the pain conditions I discuss in this book impact a sufferer's lifestyle.

CP/CPPS Treatments

The male patients I have seen come with a history of being prescribed mainly antibiotics, without successful remediation of their pain. Research literature prescribes medications for enlarged prostate including 5-ARI drugs (5-alpha reductase inhibitors), and PDE5 (phosphodiesterase-5) inhibitors for erectile dysfunction as being possibly helpful for this condition.

After taking a history and doing a physical, the patient gets the usually prescribed diet, supplements, and PEMF therapy. If that is unsuccessful, then neural trigger point therapy (as in female CPP treatment) often does the trick. The injections involved are primarily the procaine blebs in the inguinal (groin) and testicular regions only where there is pain upon palpation. The pelvic injection is a helpful one for males with symptoms of prostatitis just as it is for females with symptoms of chronic pelvic pain.

With proper training, any doctor can perform this procedure. I had a urologist once send me two patients, both with similar histories of CP and failure with standard treatments. They both came a total of three times each, then stopped coming to see me after their treatments were successful.

When I spoke to the referring urologist about what happened to them, he said one had complete recovery from his pain, and the other was 90 percent better and was happy to live with that little bit of remaining pain. Many male patients have seen me for this treatment and left without any further prostatitis symptoms. Male athletes diagnosed with this condition more often than not are actually suffering from inguinal pain and usually the residual effects from straining during workouts. The remedy is neural trigger point therapy blebs. I hope to publish a study on this condition in the future so that urologists will have more to offer to the 90 percent of their patients with CP/CPPS.

CHAPTER 13

Beyond Scars: Chronic Postoperative Pain (CPOP)

"Out of the suffering have emerged the strongest souls;
the most massive characters are seared with scars."

—Kahlil Gibran

In 2008, *The Lancet* published an estimate saying that approximately 234 million surgeries occurred annually around the world.[1] Surgery and surgeons have obviously made an enormous contribution to the practice of medicine worldwide. Unfortunately, CPOP can occur in as many as 85 percent of patients.[2] Millions of patients are affected each year and this condition can last months to years.

CPOP is pain lasting greater than three to six months after surgery. One explanation for its high prevalence is that damage is done to a major peripheral nerve by the operation. CPOP is difficult, costly, and can reduce quality of life and economic productivity for many patients. Some of the common types of CPOP I see in my practice include pain following major thoracic surgery, inguinal hernia repair, breast surgery, and orthopedic surgery.

Maggie's Story: Postoperative Abdominal Pain

"For years and years (since the eighties), I have had bouts of horrible abdominal pain from which I ended up in the hospital once or twice a year. The pain would be unendurable, and I would spend six to twelve hours throwing up and would not leave the bathroom, ending up exhausted, dehydrated, and out of it for a couple of days after.

"Whenever I ended up in the hospital or at a doctor's office for one of these episodes, they would take MRIs and other tests, yet I never had a real diagnosis. When those episodes started occurring once or twice a month, the medical establishment began running tests for Crohn's disease, gallstones, kidney stones, etc. I had colonoscopies and endoscopies, but nothing was found, except that there was a narrowing of my small intestines in one section. It was no more than five centimeters long and, in all likelihood, caused by scar tissue from past abdominal operations, of which I'd had several. The only option left was to go back and have more surgery to remove that part of the small intestine, which posed its own risks and more scar tissue possibilities. So, I needed to think about that.

"Then I met Dr. Hirani, and what she did was magical. She used neural trigger point therapy as developed by Dr. Huneke and oxygen-ozone therapy, which turned out to be the bomb! I felt like a charm again. I had not realized I was in constant pain at a level I had learned to live with. In other words, a pain level around three to five out of ten is what I was experiencing on a daily basis.

"When the attacks came on, the pain level would go up to eight or nine out of ten. At this point, I would pass out! I needed Dr. Hirani's treatment of neural trigger point and oxygen-ozone initially every two weeks for a couple of months. Then I had attacks every month that she treated each time with success. Now the attacks come about once every two to three months. She resolves the pain each time.

"I am hopeful that eventually, after enough reprogramming by the neural trigger point therapy and oxygen-ozone, my abdominal pain attacks will diminish to very little or none at all. Living with constant pain, I had not realized what a nasty person I had become around my husband and others I cared for. I was abrupt and had no patience for anything. Boy, did that change once the pain was treated by Dr. Hirani!

"I was told by my husband and others how much easier I was to get along with now. Not only did my quality of life change, but so did that of others around me—for the better, of course. It is wonderful to live life without constant pain. I am so grateful to have met Dr. Karima Hirani for many reasons. She is a wonderful human being, committed to a person's well-being by using the least invasive of procedures. My quality of life is a hundred times better since she started helping me."

Maggie is a coach in a self-development course I took a while back. One night during the course, she told the class about how she almost canceled it due to her severe pain. I offered my services to her and she jumped on it.

The first time I saw her abdomen, with all the different surgical scars from previous surgeries, I knew we were dealing with CPOP. Her previous physicians cited that the pain was likely due to scars from all these surgeries and prescribed painkillers whenever she had an attack. Ironically, the doctors had been telling her the truth about the scars. However, the common understanding when patients have pain postoperatively is they believe that the pain is only due to internal scarring from surgeries. The actual scars on the skin surface after surgery are given no importance as to the possible etiology of the pain.

The attacks were generally every two weeks when I met her. Neural trigger point therapy was first done on her, with particular regard to the scar injections, followed by neural blebs over the remaining areas of her abdomen that were tender on palpation. Once I brought in the oxygen-ozone, she experienced instant relief. It was gratifying to hear that the calmness she got from the treatment spilled into her relationships with her loved ones. Unfortunately, Maggie has not followed the recommended anti-inflammatory diet—specifically, she's failed to cut out the gluten, dairy, or sugar. She also hasn't worked on her stress reduction as much as she should. As a result, she keeps coming back for treatment. For her, this is a better alternative to further surgery and risking complications and more pain.

CPOP Treatment

Many factors are at play in the development of CPOP. They include genetics, psychological states, pre-existing pain, individual inflammatory response to tissue damage, and surgical technique as well as the anesthesia.

Inguinal hernia surgery can leave about 29 to 43 percent of patients with moderate to severe chronic pain.[3] Inguinal hernias are more common in men than women.[4] Even sex can become painful. CPOP is the most common and severe long-term problem in men after hernia repair.

After breast surgeries like mastectomies, 20 to 50 percent of women experience CPOP.[5] They can have scar pain, phantom breast pain, or other pain. There is a condition called postmastectomy pain syndrome. In one Scottish longitudinal study that looked at women postmastectomy and three years postoperatively, 50 percent continued to suffer from pain up to twelve years after surgery.[6]

The pain management for these patients has not been very successful. NSAIDs or Tylenol® and, if necessary, opioid medications and anticonvulsants (e.g., Neurontin®) are common medications given. My usual protocol is employed for these patients when they come to see me. The surgical scars can be a considerable interference field and source of pain; they must, first and foremost, be treated with the procaine injection just underneath the scar (see Chapter 5 scar treatment discussion and photo).

Tender points or trigger points must be sought out through a careful palpation technique and subsequently injected with procaine blebs. If necessary, I will use oxygen-ozone to bring about either improvement or complete resolution of the pain. The PEMF therapy can work to lower the pain level[7] and so can the anti-inflammatory diet and supplements. PRP therapy has been used to treat scars from burn pain.[8]

The Role of Stress

Stress seems to play a big role in pain such as in Maggie's case, which confirms researchers' conclusions that CPOP is multifactorial in its origin, and the psychological state is one of those factors. I cannot emphasize enough the need for all chronic pain suffers to address their stress and anxiety. Neural trigger point therapy in the abdominal area is thought to treat the adrenal glands and brings about a calm state for the patient, which can last for days, weeks, or months.

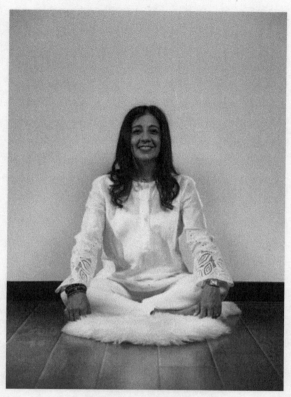

Dr. Hirani doing her daily Kundalini yoga, which helps with stress reduction.

If you are a CPOP sufferer, it is essential to look at your level of stress, your diet, and your exercise level. If there is any deficiency in these areas, start with correcting them on your own at first. Try the anti-inflammatory diet and take some supplements I discussed in Chapter 3. Then, find a way to reduce your stress. Maggie is so grateful she has her life back and doesn't have to live in fear of the next attack. I have successfully treated hundreds of patients like her.

CHAPTER 14

Tips on Taking Your Journey to Freedom from Pain

"Pain can change you, but never let it define you."

—Heidi Rader

There is a lot that your doctor didn't tell you about your pain. Contrary to the standard line that's given to patients, *you can achieve greater than just 50 percent improvement* in your pain. After reading this book, you should recognize how you and your doctors have been manipulated through mass media marketing and persuasion. The bottom line is that you've been sold a bill of goods that pain medications are mostly all that is available to treat your pain and that you will most likely never receive anything resembling a complete recovery.

We talked about how there is no profit if you don't continue to hurt. If something like diet and exercise can bring about 25 to 30 percent improvement in pain alone, yet this isn't marketed to doctors or patients alike, how can we expect PEMF therapy, neural trigger point therapy, or oxygen-ozone therapy to become widely known? As discussed, these alternative modalities of treatment are not going to drive huge revenues. If you just follow the course prescribed by advertisers and conventional medicine, your pain will most likely never go away.

Your pain doesn't have to be perpetual. It can be treated. Your stress and anxiety, loss of income, and affected relationships don't have to keep you in a prison of life-long pain.

Please see the two next images for my top ten list of some simple things you can do right now to manage your pain.

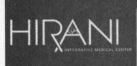

TOP 10 TIPS TO MANAGE PAIN

Learn More

www.drhirani.com

1 Change your diet!

Try the elimination diet or get tested for IgG and IgE food allergies and sensitivities.

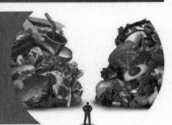

2 Exercise!

Start with a short five-minute walk daily, then gradually increase to an hour a day. Ask for a physical therapy prescription.

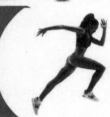

3 Stop smoking!

The role that smoking plays in many chronic and deadly diseases is well established.

4 Eat omega-3 fats!

You can get these from eating fish or supplements.

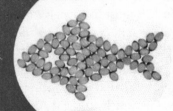

5 Get your vitamin D every day

Consume it as a vitamin D3 supplement or get it from sunshine.

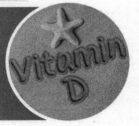

6 Take magnesium & B12 for headaches

Ask your doctor for a shot of these two amazing substances. And if she won't prescribe you the injection, then take it orally.

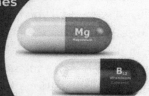

7 Reduce your stress & anxiety now!

There are plenty of great solutions (Kundalini yoga is what works for me). Please don't ignore it. This is the number one contributor to chronic illness.

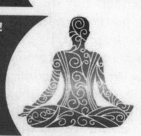

8 Earth-based PEMFs

Sit outside in the sunshine daily, ideally barefoot on the ground for an hour a day (you can make vitamin D at the same time).

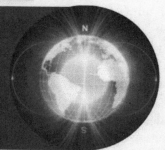

9 PEMF therapy

Try the two types: both the high and low intensity.

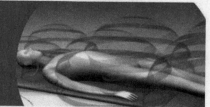

10 Educate yourself on neural trigger point therapy & oxygen-ozone therapy

Find a worthy practitioner as not every doctor trained in neural trigger point therapy or oxygen-ozone therapy performs it the same.

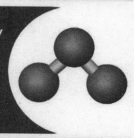

If you have tried all of the above recommendations as well as PRP and UC-MSCs, and if you found no relief for your pain, *please don't give up hope.* I would be lying to you if I said I have a 100 percent success rate with all pain patients.

When I don't succeed, I always ask them: "Are you following all of my recommendations including diet, supplements, exercise, and stress reduction?" It is often when a patient refuses to make dietary changes or work on their stress, that keeps them coming back for more treatments or results in a lack of success. Of course, I do have patients who have followed all my recommendations and yet still have their pain. In these cases, we have to go beyond the treatments discussed in this book. I would sincerely like to hear from readers about what has helped you the most.

As I am writing this book, I have started training in musculoskeletal ultrasound–guided injections. An area of great fascination to me is the hydrodissection of nerves under ultrasound guidance. The procedure involves using a solution of anesthetic like procaine along with sugar water to gently lift the irritating nerve/nerve root, and thereby bring about significant pain relief.

For such unresponsive patients as cited above, this also means taking a deeper look into the mechanism of chronic illness. Is there an autoimmune, nutritional deficiency, hormonal, or environmental component that is triggering your chronic pain? My mentor once said, "Have you done everything you can possibly do for your patient? If not, then your work is not done." *As long as there is hope, I am committed to searching for alternative pain solutions.*

For more information visit www.drhirani.com. And please follow me on Facebook and LinkedIn.

ON PAIN
BY KHALIL GIBRAN,
FROM *THE PROPHET*

Your pain is the breaking of the shell that encloses your understanding.

Even as the stone of the fruit must break, that its heart may stand in the sun, so must you know pain.

And could you keep your heart in wonder at the daily miracles of your life, your pain would not seem less wondrous than your joy;

And you would accept the seasons of your heart even as you have always accepted the seasons that pass over your fields.

And you would watch with serenity through the winters of your grief.

Much of your pain is self-chosen.

It is the bitter potion by which the physician within you heals your sick self.

Therefore, trust the physician, and drink his remedy in silence and tranquility:

For his hand, though heavy and hard, is guided by the tender hand of the Unseen,

And the cup he brings, though it burn your lips, has been fashioned of the clay which the Potter has moistened with His own sacred tears.

Appendices

Select Abbreviations, Acronyms, and Initialisms

AD-MSC	adipose-derived mesenchymal stem cells
BM-MCS	bone marrow-derived mesenchymal stem cells
CAM	complementary and alternative medicine
CBT	cognitive behavioral therapy
CIM	complementary and integrative medicine
CP/CPPS	chronic prostatitis/chronic pelvic pain syndrome
CPOP	chronic postoperative pain
CPP	chronic pelvic pain
DPN	diabetic peripheral neuropathy
GI	gastrointestinal
IBS	irritable bowel syndrome
IgE	immunoglobulin E
IgG	immunoglobulin G
IV	intravenous
LBP	low back pain
LDA	low-dose allergen
LDN	low-dose naltrexone
MS	multiple sclerosis

MSCs	mesenchymal stem cells
NSAIDs	nonsteroidal anti-inflammatory drugs
PEMF	pulsed electromagnetic field
PHN	postherpetic neuralgia
PRP	platelet-rich plasma
SCD	sickle cell disease
TMJ	temporomandibular joint
TTH	tension-type headache
UC-MSCs	umbilical cord-derived mesenchymal stem cells

Glossary

Acupuncture:

Originating in China, an integrative medicine treatment (with similar principles to neural trigger point therapy) for which very thin needles are applied to areas on the body to restore the Chi or energy flow.

Acute:

Of new onset and opposite of chronic.

Aerobic exercise:

Brisk exercise (e.g., running, swimming, bicycling) that promotes the circulation of oxygen through the blood and is associated with an increased rate of breathing.

Adipose tissue:

A specialized connective tissue consisting of fat-rich cells (adipocytes) that makes up 20 to 25 percent of total body weight in healthy individuals.

Adrenal glands:

Small, triangular-shaped glands that sit above both kidneys and produce hormones to regulate metabolism, the immune system, blood pressure, response to stress, and other functions.

Analgesia:

Loss of pain sensation.

Anticonvulsant medication:

Diverse group of pharmacological drugs primarily intended to treat seizure disorders, but which have been used in treatment of bipolar disorder and neuropathic pain.

Antioxidant:

A compound that has an extra electron that it can donate to a free radical (unstable molecule that causes oxidative stress), thereby stabilizing it and preventing damage to cells in the body.

Antispasmodic drug:

A pharmaceutical drug that reduces muscle spasms.

Antidepressant medication:

A prescription drug used to treat major depression, anxiety, and some chronic pain conditions.

Aquatic:

Relating to water.

Autologous:

Cells or tissue obtained from the same individual being treated.

Aura:

Sensation (e.g., flashing lights, a gleam of light, blurred vision, an odor, the feeling of a breeze, numbness, weakness, difficulty in speaking) perceived by a patient just before onset of a seizure or migraine.

Ayurvedic medicine:

The world's oldest holistic healing systems (developed more than three thousand years ago in India), which is founded on the belief that health and wellness depend on a delicate balance between mind, body, and spirit.

B12:

A water-soluble vitamin found in liver, meat, eggs, poultry, shellfish, milk, and milk products that the body needs to help make red blood cells, DNA, RNA, energy, and tissues as well as to keep nerve cells healthy.

Bleb:

A small bubble or blister on the skin that is filled with fluid.

Bone marrow:

A soft, fatty substance in the center of bones in which blood cells and stem cells are produced.

BM-MSCs:

Bone marrow–derived mesenchymal stem cells.

Bone spur:

Bony growth that develops on the edge of a bone, which can cause symptoms of pain as it is pushing up against your nerves, tendons, or muscles.

Brain fog:

A term used for certain symptoms that can affect your ability to think (e.g., confusion, disorganized thoughts, difficulty focusing or putting thoughts into words).

Bursa:

A fluid-filled sac or saclike cavity, which acts as a cushion and gliding surface countering friction between tissues of the body.

Cardiovascular:

Pertaining to the heart and blood vessels.

Cellular differentiation:

Process in which a cell changes from one cell type (immature) to another type (specialized).

Cartilage:

Firm, whitish, flexible connective tissue found in various forms and locations (e.g., surfaces of joints).

Central nervous system:

Consists of the brain and spinal cord, which is a complex of nerve tissues to control the activities of the body.

Cervical spine:

Neck region consisting of seven bones (vertebrae) separated from each other by discs.

Chemotherapy:

A type of cancer treatment that uses one or more anticancer drugs as part of a standardized chemotherapy regimen.

Chinese medicine:

A medical system used for thousands of years to prevent, diagnose, and treat disease, which holds that the body's vital energy, or Chi, flows along meridians (channels) in the body and helps keep a person balanced in spiritual, emotional, mental, and physical health.

CP/CPPS:

Chronic prostatitis/chronic pelvic pain syndrome.

CPOP:

Chronic postoperative pain.

CPP:

Chronic pelvic pain.

Cognitive behavioral therapy (CBT):

A psychosocial intervention that aims to improve mental health and well-being.

Complementary and alternative medicine (CAM):

Term used to describe the practice that is used either together with (complementary) or instead of (alternative to) standard medical care (e.g., megadose vitamins, herbs, acupuncture, PEMF, neural trigger point therapy, oxygen-ozone therapy).

Compounded drug:

A process of combining, mixing, or altering ingredients to create a medication tailored to the needs of an individual patient.

Compounding pharmacy:

A specialty pharmacy that makes prescription medications from scratch (not mass-produced or one-size-fits-all formulations).

Cortisol:

A steroid hormone that regulates a wide range of processes throughout the body (e.g., metabolism, immune response) and that has a vital role in helping the body respond to stress.

Dairy:

A food that is made from a mammal's milk (e.g., cow, goat, sheep, camel).

Dermatome:

Area of the skin that is supplied by nerves from a single spinal nerve root.

Diabetic peripheral neuropathy (DPN):

Nerve damage seen in diabetes that affects the legs and feet which can be painful, debilitating, and fatal.

Differentiation:

See cellular differentiation.

Disc:

Fibrocartilage that lies between the adjacent vertebrae in the spinal column, allowing for slight movement of the vertebrae and functioning as a shock absorber for the spine.

Double-blind study:

Research study where neither the patients nor the researchers know who is receiving the actual treatment versus the placebo, thereby preventing bias when doctors evaluate patient outcomes and improving reliability of the study.

Dyspareunia:

Pain or difficulty with intercourse.

Epstein-Barr virus:

A herpes virus causing infectious mononucleosis and associated with fatigue, fever, lack of appetite, rash, sore throat, swollen glands in the neck, weakness, and sore muscles.

Edema:

A swelling caused by excess fluid trapped in your body's tissues.

Empathy:

The ability to put yourself in another's shoes, feeling or understanding what another person is feeling or going through.

Endometriosis:

A painful disorder in which tissue that normally lines the uterus grows outside of the uterus.

Enzyme:

A biological catalyst that helps to speed up a biochemical reaction in the body.

Epidural injection:

Usually, a steroid injection with anesthetic delivered into the epidural space to help reduce inflammation and pain.

Epidural space:

An anatomic space located in the spinal canal between the spinal dura matter (membrane) and the vertebral column.

Fanconi syndrome:

A disorder of kidney tubes in which certain substances normally absorbed back into the bloodstream by the kidneys are lost into the urine instead.

Fascia:

A covering of every structure of the body, creating a structural continuity that gives form and function to every tissue and organ.

Fibromyalgia:

A chronic disorder with widespread musculoskeletal pain, fatigue, and tenderness in localized areas.

Flavonoids:

Phytonutrients found in almost all fruits and vegetables (giving these their vivid colors) that function as powerful antioxidants with anti-inflammatory and immune system benefits.

Frankenhauser plexus:

A group of autonomic nerves on either side of the cervix.

Free radical:

Uncharged molecule having an uneven number of electrons and which is unstable and can cause damage to your cells.

Frozen shoulder:

A stiffness and pain in the shoulder joint, which can take up to three years to resolve.

Gluten:

A substance present in many cereal grains that is composed of primarily two classes of proteins, gliadin and glutenin, and can cause illness in people with celiac disease and sensitivity or intolerance in other patients.

Groin:

Inguinal region of the body located between the abdomen (belly) and the thigh on either side of the body.

Growth factor:

A naturally occurring substance—usually a secreted protein or steroid hormone—capable of stimulating cell proliferation, wound healing, and occasionally cellular differentiation.

G6PD deficiency:

An inherited condition causing red blood cells to break down in response to certain medications, infections, or other stressors.

Hemorrhagic condition:

Bleeding disorder that is excessive or abnormal.

Herniated disc:

A problem with one of the rubbery cushions (discs) that sit between the individual bones (vertebrae) that stack to make your spine, wherein the soft center of the disc pushes through its tougher exterior.

Hyaluronic acid injection:

Helps the fluid in your joints, treating knee pain caused by osteoarthritis in patients who have failed with traditional pain relievers and other treatments.

Hyperthyroidism:

Overactive thyroid, which occurs when the thyroid gland overproduces thyroid hormone.

IgE antibody:

Immunoglobulin E, an antibody produced by the immune system in response to an allergen, causing a reaction that can be immediate (e.g., hives; throat, tongue, or mouth swelling; asthmatic presentation).

IgG antibody:

Immunoglobulin G, a type of antibody that makes up 75 percent of circulating antibodies, the main role of which is to protect you from reinfection from a virus or bacterium, but also present as a response to exposure to foods (pain, fatigue, depression), which can appear hours or days later.

IgG food antibody test:

Test for food sensitivity, where blood is drawn and tested with food components, and the degree of IgG antibody binding to the foods is quantified and reported (not the same as testing for food allergies, and there exists controversy on validity of this test).

Iliopsoas bursitis:

Inflammation (caused by arthritis, trauma, or infection) of the largest bursa in the body, which is located beneath the iliopsoas muscle or between the front of the hip joint and the hip flexor muscle.

Immune system:

A complex network of cells, tissues, and organs (including white blood cells and the lymphatic system), producing substances to help the body fight infections and other diseases.

Inguinal:

Of, related to, or situated in the groin area.

Integrative medicine:

The combination of mainstream medicine with the best of evidence-based alternative medicine.

Interference field:

In neural trigger point therapy, any trauma, infection, or surgery can damage a portion of the autonomic nervous system and produce longstanding disturbances in the electrochemical or electromagnetic functions of these tissues.

Intra-articular injection:

Joint injection.

Intradermal injection:

An injection that goes between the layers of the skin (superficial).

Intramuscular injection:

An injection administered into a muscle.

Intravenous injection:

An injection administered into a vein (e.g., intravenous drip).

Irritable bowel syndrome (IBS):

A widespread disorder involving recurrent abdominal pain and diarrhea or constipation, often associated with stress, depression, anxiety, or previous infection.

Lifestyle modification:

Involves altering long-standing habits of eating or physical activity and maintaining the new behavior for months or years to treat diseases like obesity and pain.

Low-dose allergy (LDA) therapy:

A safe, effective homeopathic or micro-dosing remedy used to treat food and environmental allergies as well as autoimmune conditions, which can be administered sublingually (under the tongue).

Low-dose naltrexone:

An off-label, experimental use of the medication naltrexone at low doses to help regulate a dysfunctional immune system.

Lumbar spine:

Lower back, consisting of five vertebrae in the lower part of the spine.

Lyme disease:

An inflammatory disease (e.g., rash, headache, fever, chills, arthritis, neurological disorders, cardiac disorders) that is caused by the bacteria *Borrelia burgdorferi*, which is transmitted by a blacklegged tick, a.k.a. deer tick (although these ticks are not limited to deer).

Lymphatic system:

An organ system that is part of the circulatory system and the immune system, the vessels of which carry lymph or waste from the cells for removal.

Magnesium:

An abundant mineral in the body, naturally present in many foods and a cofactor in more than three hundred enzyme reactions in the body, which has been shown to helpful in neurological disorders and in shutting off the pain stimulus.

MSCs:

Mesenchymal stem cells.

Metabolite:

An intermediate or end product of metabolism, which is usually a smaller molecule compared to the original compound.

Menstruation:

The normal vaginal bleeding that occurs every month in a woman of childbearing age, aka her "period."

Mindfulness-based cognitive therapy (MBCT):

A modified form of CBT that incorporates CBT together with meditation and breathing exercises to break away from negative thought patterns that can cause a downward spiral in mental and physical well-being.

Multipotent stem cell:

Cells that have the capacity to self-renew by dividing and to develop into multiple specialized cell types present in a specific damaged tissue.

Muscle spasticity:

A condition in which the muscles stiffen or tighten, preventing normal movement, as seen in MS.

Mutation:

The changing of the structure of a gene, resulting in a variation of the DNA that can be transmitted to subsequent generations.

Multiple myeloma:

A cancer of plasma cells (a type of white blood cell) in the bone marrow, the spread of which can cause damage and pain to the bones, immune system, kidneys, and red blood cell count.

Multiple sclerosis (MS):

A potentially disabling disease of the brain and spinal cord, where the immune system is targeting the myelin sheath (the tissue that surrounds your nerves).

Myofascial:

Relating to the fascia surrounding and separating muscle tissue.

Narcotic pain medicine (aka opioid pain relievers):

Derivatives of opium.

Nonsteroidal anti-inflammatory drug (NSAID):

A medication in a drug class that reduces pain, decreases fever, prevents blood clots, and (in high doses) decreases inflammation.

Nerve block:

The production of loss of sensation or pain in a part of the body by injecting an anesthetic near the nerves that supply it.

Nerve root (fiber):

Initial segment of a nerve leaving the central nervous system (brain stem or spinal cord).

Neural trigger point therapy:

See Chapter 5.

Neuron:

Specialized cell or nerve cell that transmits nerve impulses or signals.

Neuropathic pain:

Pain caused by a lesion or disease of the somatosensory nervous system.

Novocain:

Another name for procaine.

Osteoarthritis:

Degeneration of joint cartilage and the underlying bone, most common from middle age onward, causing pain and stiffness, especially in the hip, knee, and thumb joints.

Osteoporosis:

A condition in which the bones become weak, brittle, and fragile due to loss of tissue, potentially resulting in bone fractures.

Ovarian cyst:

Solid or fluid-filled sac or pocket within or on the surface of the ovary.

Oxygen-ozone therapy:

See Chapter 6.

Oxidative stress:

An imbalance between free radicals and antioxidants (see definitions on preceding pages) in your body.

Oxidizing agent:

A chemical substance that causes another chemical substance to lose electrons and then become unstable like a free radical.

Palpation:

The process of using one's hands to check the body to diagnose a disease or illness.

Paraspinal injections:

Injection in the muscles that keep your spine erect (the erector spinae).

Peri-axillary:

Adjacent to the armpit.

Peripheral nerve:

Part of the nervous system consisting of nerves outside of the brain and spinal cord.

Pes anserine bursitis:

Inflammation of the bursa located between the shinbone (tibia) and three tendons of the hamstring muscle at the inside of the knee.

Phantom limb pain:

Perception of pain or discomfort in a limb that no longer exists (due to amputation).

Phantom breast pain:

Perception of pain or discomfort in a breast that has been removed (usually due to breast cancer).

Pharmacological:

Pertaining to prescription drugs.

Physical therapy:

The treatment of disease, injury, or deformity by physical methods such as massage, heat treatment, and exercise rather than with drugs or surgery.

Phytonutrients:

A broad name for a variety of compounds produced by plants (e.g., fruits, vegetables, beans, grains) that can improve your health.

Placebo-controlled study:

A way of testing a medical therapy by giving one group of patients the actual therapy/treatment and the other group a placebo (or sham) therapy/treatment that has no real effect.

Platelet-rich plasma (PRP) therapy:

Post-herpetic neuralgia: Most common complication of shingles or herpes zoster, affecting the nerve fibers and skin and causing burning pain that lasts long after the rash and blisters of shingles disappear.

Post-mastectomy syndrome:

Type of chronic neuropathic pain disorder that occurs following breast cancer surgeries.

Prana:

Breath or life-giving force of energy that flows in currents in and around the body.

Premenstrual syndrome:

A group of symptoms (e.g., mood swings, painful breasts, abdominal [belly] cramps, depression, fatigue) in women that occurs between ovulation and a period.

Procaine (aka Novocaine):

Synthetic compound derived from benzoic acid and used as a local anesthetic, especially in dentistry.

Progesterone:

Sex hormone involved in the menstrual cycle and pregnancy and which may be responsible for migraine headaches in women.

Pubic symphis:

Cartilaginous joint between the left and right pubic bones near the midline of the body, above any external genitals and in front of the bladder.

Pulsed electromagnetic field (PEMF) therapy:

Use of electromagnetic fields to attempt to heal damaged tissues and relieve pain.

Radiculopathy:

A disease of the root of the nerve, such as from a pinched nerve or a tumor, which can cause a lot of pain (e.g., sciatica).

Randomized study:

A scientific experiment that aims to reduce bias by randomly allocating the patients (by chance) to either receive the treatment or the placebo.

Receptor:

A specialized molecular structure that sits on the cell surface or inside it and that binds with substances such as hormones, drugs, or neurotransmitters.

Regenerative medicine:

A branch of medicine that deals with the process of replacing cells and tissue to restore or establish normal function.

Restless leg syndrome:

An uncontrollable urge to move your legs, typically happening in the evening or nighttime when you're sitting or lying down.

Rheumatoid arthritis:

A chronic progressive disease that causes inflammation in the joints, resulting in painful deformities as well as immobility, especially in the fingers, wrists, feet, and ankles.

Rotator cuff tendinitis:

Irritation of the tendons of shoulder muscles (rotator cuff muscles) and inflammation of the bursa lining the tendons.

Sacral spine:

A large triangular bone at the base of the spine that forms by fusing of sacral vertebrae.

Saline:

A solution of salt in water, which can be given intravenously.

Sepsis:

A potentially life-threatening complication of an infection that has spread throughout the body and can manifest with symptoms such as fever, difficulty breathing, low blood pressure, fast heart rate, and confusion.

Shin:

The front of the leg below the knee, which is a common area of pain (shin splint).

Shingles (aka herpes zoster):

A reactivation of the chickenpox (varicella) virus in the body that causes a painful rash, involving acute painful inflammation along the nerve root.

Sickle cell anemia:

A severe hereditary form of anemia (most common among those of African descent) in which hemoglobin in red blood cells cannot carry as much oxygen and the atypical hemoglobin distorts the red blood cells into a crescent (sickle) shape.

Sickle shape:

Crescent shape of red blood cells due to atypical hemoglobin molecules distorting red blood cells in sickle cell disease.

Sinus:

A cavity within a bone of the face or skull connecting with nasal cavities, which is often a site of pain and headaches.

Skeletal muscle:

A muscle that is connected to the skeleton to form part of the mechanical system which moves the limbs and other parts of the body.

Sleep apnea:

A potentially serious sleep disorder in which breathing repeatedly stops and starts.

Soft tissue:

Tissue that is not hardened or calcified (e.g., tendons, muscles, skin, fat, fascia).

Spine (aka backbone):

A series of vertebrae that extend from the skull to the small of the back (i.e., where the spine curves at the end of the waist), enclosing the spinal cord and providing support for the thorax and abdomen.

Somatosensory nervous system:

A part of the sensory nervous system that is a complex system of sensory neurons and neural pathways and which responds to changes at the surface or inside the body.

Subcutaneous injection:

An injection just underneath the skin.

Tendon:

A flexible (but inelastic) cord of strong fibrous collagen tissue attaching a muscle to a bone.

Tendinosis (tendinopathy):

Degeneration of the tendon's collagen in response to chronic overuse.

Tension-type headache:

A diffuse, mild-to-moderate pain in your head that is often described as feeling like having a tight band around your head.

Thrombocytopenia:

Deficiency of platelets in the blood, causing bleeding into tissues, bruising, and slow blood clotting after injury.

Temporomandibular joint dysfunction (aka TMJ):

Pain and compromised movement of the jaw joint and surrounding muscles.

Transcranial magnetic stimulation (TMS):

A noninvasive form of brain stimulation in which a changing magnetic field (PEMF) is used to activate an electric current at a specific area of the brain.

Transcutaneous electrical nerve stimulation (TENS):

Uses electrical currents across the intact surface of the skin to activate underlying nerves to bring about pain relief.

Trapezius muscle:

A large, flat, triangular, superficial muscle on each side of the neck.

Trigger point:

A sensitive area in the muscle or connective tissue (fascia) that becomes painful when compressed.

Umbilical cord:

A flexible, cordlike structure containing blood vessels and other tissue that attaches the developing fetus to the mother's placenta, thereby deriving nutrients from her.

UC-MSCs:

Umbilical cord-derived mesenchymal stem cells.

Uterine fibroid:

Benign growth in the uterus that can develop during a woman's childbearing years.

Zoster (aka herpes zoster or shingles):

Caused by the reactivation of the varicella zoster virus along the dermatomes, causing a rash that can be very painful.

Helpful Resources and Additional Literature References

Books About Diet and Pain

The Complete Anti-Inflammatory Diet for Beginners: A No-Stress Meal Plan with Easy Recipes to Heal the Immune System by Dorothy Calimeris and Lulu Cook, RDN

Plant Based Diet for Chronic Pain by Emily George

The Complete Mediterranean Cookbook: 500 Vibrant, Kitchen-Tested Recipes for Living and Eating Well Every Day by America's Test Kitchen

Books About Fitness

Balance & Strength Exercises for Seniors: 9 Practices, with Traditional Exercises, and Modified Tai Chi, Yoga & Dance Based Movements by Jane Adams

Becoming a Supple Leopard (2nd ed.): The Ultimate Guide to Resolving Pain, Preventing Injury, and Optimizing Athletic Performance by Dr. Kelly Starrett with Glen Cordoza

Tai Chi Fit: Over 50 Beginner Exercises with David-Dorian Ross by David-Dorian Ross

Neural Therapy

Manual of Neural Therapy According to Huneke (2nd ed.) by Mathias Dosch, MD, and Peter Dosch, MD.

"Neural Therapy" by Michael Gurevich, MD: https://www.brmi.online/post/neural-therapy

Manual of Neural Therapy According to Huneke: Therapy with Local Anesthetics
(11th ed.) by Peter Dosch, MD
*Facts about Neural Therapy according to Huneke: (Regulating Therapy) Brief
Summary for Patients* by Wilhelma Dosch

Oxygen-Ozone Therapy

Articles about oxygen-ozone therapy: https://www.brmi.online/articles-
oxygen-ozone-therapy
*The Ozone Miracle: How you can harness the power of oxygen to keep you and
your family healthy* by Frank Shallenberger MD, HMD

PEMF Therapy

PEMF Advisor: www.pemfadvisor.com

PRP Therapy

OrthoInfo from the American Academy of Orthopaedic Surgeons:
Orthoinfo.aaos.org/en/treatment/platelet-rich-plasma-prp
*The Book on PRP: An easy to understand "consumer's guide" to understanding
how platelet-rich plasma is used to treat problems such as tendonitis,
bursitis, and other related disorders* by Nathan Wei, MD

Stem Cell Therapy

*The Healing Revolution: Chronic Pain Relief and Regeneration without Drugs
or Surgery* by Dr. Raj Banerjee
PromoCell: Promocell.com/blog/using-mesenchymal-stem-cells-in-
regenerative-medicine/

Websites

National Center for Complementary and Integrative Health: nccih.nih.gov/
health/pain
Integrative Pain Science Institute: integrativepainscienceinstitute.com

Journal Articles

Diet / headache

Razeghi Jahromi, S., Ghorbani, Z., Martelletti, P. *et al*. Association of diet and headache. *J Headache Pain* 20, 106 (2019). https://doi.org/10.1186/ s10194-019-1057-1

PEMF / pelvic pain

Jorgensen, W. A., Frome, B. M., & Wallach, C. (1994). Electrochemical therapy of pelvic pain: effects of pulsed electromagnetic fields (PEMF) on tissue trauma. *The European journal of surgery. Supplement.: = Acta chirurgica. Supplement*, (574), 83–86.

PEMF / rheumatoid arthritis and fibromyalgia

Shupak, N. M., McKay, J. C., Nielson, W. R., Rollman, G. B., Prato, F. S., & Thomas, A. W. (2006). Exposure to a Specific Pulsed Low-Frequency Magnetic Field: A Double-Blind Placebo-Controlled Study of Effects on Pain Ratings in Rheumatoid Arthritis and Fibromyalgia Patients. *Pain Research and Management*, *11*(2), 85–90. https://doi. org/10.1155/2006/842162

PRP / shoulder pain

Rha, D. W., Park, G. Y., Kim, Y. K., Kim, M. T., & Lee, S. C. (2013). Comparison of the therapeutic effects of ultrasound-guided platelet-rich plasma injection and dry needling in rotator cuff disease: a randomized controlled trial. *Clinical rehabilitation*, *27*(2), 113–122. https://doi. org/10.1177/0269215512448388

Stem cells / neuropathic pain

Yousefifard, M., Nasirinezhad, F., Shardi Manaheji, H. *et al*. Human bone marrow-derived and umbilical cord-derived mesenchymal stem cells for alleviating neuropathic pain in a spinal cord injury model. *Stem Cell Res Ther* 7, 36 (2016). https://doi.org/10.1186/s13287-016-0295-2

Stem cells / spinal cord injury

Yang, C., Wang, G., Ma, F., Yu, B., Chen, F., Yang, J., Feng, J., & Wang, Q. (2018). Repeated injections of human umbilical cord blood-derived mesenchymal stem cells significantly promote functional recovery in rabbits with spinal cord injury of two noncontinuous segments. *Stem cell research & therapy*, *9*(1), 136. https://doi.org/10.1186/s13287-018-0879-0

Neural Therapy Timeline

Frank, B. L. (1999). "Neural Therapy." *Physical Medicine and Rehabilitation Clinics of North America*, *10*(3), 573–582. https://doi.org/10.1016/s1047-9651(18)30181-5

(This timeline, which appears on pages 573–574, is shared below with kind permission from timeline author Bryan L. Frank, MD.)

Historical Perspectives

Neural therapy has its origins in numerous discoveries throughout medical history that have furthered understanding of pain, cutaneous reflexes, local anesthetics, and the autonomic nervous system. A short list includes[4, 7-9]:

ca. 3000 BC – Chinese begin development of acupuncture theses that recognize response of pain and illness to stimulation of skin points.

1890 – Schleich performs first surgery using "infiltration anesthesia" with 0.1% cocaine solution.

1893 – Sigmund Freud discovers topical cocaine effects.

1898 – Head publishes his "Sensory Disturbances of the Skin in Visceral Diseases," which leads to understanding of cutaneovisceral reflexes.

1903 – Cathelin performs first caudal epidural injection using cocaine.

1905 – Einhorn discovers Novocain, generically known as procaine.

1906 – Speiss discovers greatly enhanced wound healing after regional infiltration with Novocain.

1906 – Vishnevski confirms the anti-inflammatory effects of locally applied Novocain.

1925 – Leriche performs first stellate ganglion block using Novocain. He describes the use of Novocain as "the surgeon's bloodless knife."

1926 – Ferdinand Huneke uses intravenous injection of procaine and cures chronic migraine headaches, which had resisted all other therapeutic endeavors for years.

1928 – Ferdinand and Walter Huneke publish "Unfamiliar Remote Effects of Local Anesthetics," based on their experiences with injection of local anesthetics in head's zones for a variety of painful conditions.[4] Kibler suggests the term "segmental therapy."

1940 – F. Huneke injects an itchy osteomyelitis scar on a patient's lower leg and immediately a previously intractable shoulder pain is cured. This is the first observed "lightning reaction" or "Huneke Phenomenon."[4]

1940 – Sieger studies allergic phenomena in animals and discovers that subcutaneous infiltration of Novocain prevents allergic reaction in subsequent exposure of allergen. He challenges the understanding of allergic responses and antibody reactions to include "tissue memory," which the local anesthetic injection erases, in addition to the antibody formation.[7]

1947 – Scheit publishes "The Autonomic System" and recognizes "interference fields" which apply to all disturbed autonomic tissues.

1951 – Ratschow tests neural therapy on 1011 cases with dramatic positive results despite poor training by the technicians administering the therapy. Ratschow observes 72 "lightning reactions."

1952 – W. Huneke publishes "Impletol Therapy and Other Neural-therapeutic Methods" in German.[4]

1961 – F. Huneke publishes "The Lightning Reaction. A Physician's Testament."

1965 – Pischinger succeeded in showing objective evidence of the lightning reaction using hematological analysis and iodometry. He advances the understanding of autonomic regulation and the relationship between the cell and the extracellular environment.[12]

1984 – Peter Dosch first publishes "Manual of Neural Therapy According to Huneke" in English (First German edition in 1964).

Citations from Dr. Frank's paper as referred to above:

4. Dosch P: Manual of neural therapy according to Huneke: Regulating therapy with local anesthetics, ed 11. Heidelbeg, Karl F. Haug Publishers, 1984

7. Klinghardt D: Neural therapy. Journal of Neurological and Orthopaedic Medicine and Surgery 14:109-114, 1993

8. Klinghardt D: Neural therapy course A: The intensive. Santa Fe, NM, Course Syllabus, 1993

9. Klinghardt D: Neural therapy course B: The neurology of the autonomic nervous system. Course Syllabus, 1993
12. Pischinger A: Matrix and Matrix Regulation, Basis for a Holistic Theory in Medicine. Brussels, Belgium, Haug International, 1991

Neural Trigger Point Therapy: Lymphatic System Theory

Bryan L. Frank, MD, also notes in his same article as above (pp. 580–581) that "in the 1970s, Fleckenstein showed that the injection of Novocain into lymphatic vessels or nodes led to the dilation of the lymphatic vessels and increased the speed of transport of lymph through the entire lymphatic system. Chronic spasm of the lymphatics may exist for long periods from injury or illness, and local anesthetic injections likely open the channels and resume normal lymphatic flow."

Endnotes

Chapter 1

1   Elin Dysvik and Bodil Furnes. "Living a meaningful life with chronic pain—further follow-up," *Clinical Case Reports*, 6(5) (2018): 896–900, https://doi.org/10.1002/ccr3.1487
2   Ibid.
3   James Dahlhamer, PhD, et al. "Prevalence of Chronic Pain and High-Impact Chronic Pain Among Adults—United States, 2016," Centers for Disease Control and Prevention, September 16 ,2018, https://www.cdc.gov/mmwr/volumes/67/wr/mm6736a2.htm
4   Ibid.

Chapter 2

1   M. Shahbandeh. "Leading U.S. Analgesic Tablet Brands 2019," Statista, September 13, 2019, https://Www.Statista.Com/Statistics/194510/Leading-Us-Analgesic-Tablet-Brands-in-2013-Based-on-Sales/.
2   Beth Snyder Bulik. "The top 10 ad spenders in Big Pharma for 2020." Fierce Pharma, April 2021, https://www.fiercepharma.com/special-report/top-10-ad-spenders-big-pharma-for-2020.
3   Ana Swanson. "Big pharmaceutical companies are spending far more on marketing than research," *Washington Post*, February 2015, https://www.washingtonpost.com/news/wonk/wp/2015/02/11/big-pharmaceutical-companies-are-spending-far-more-on-marketing-than-research/; A. Guttmann. "Pharma and healthcare industry advertising in the U.S. - statistics & facts," Statista, September 2021,
    https://www.statista.com/topics/8415/pharma-and-healthcare-industry-advertising-in-the-us/#dossierKeyfigures.
4   "Understanding the Epidemic," Centers for Disease Control and Prevention, March 19, 2020, www.cdc.gov/drugoverdose/epidemic/index.html

Chapter 3

1   Binbin Lin, et al. "Gut microbiota regulates neuropathic pain: potential mechanisms and therapeutic strategy," *Journal of Headache and Pain*, 2020; 21(1) (August 17, 2020):103. https://www.ncbi.nlm.nih.gov/pmc/articles/PMC7433133/

[2]   Zoë Dworsky-Fried, Bradley J. Kerr, and Anna M. W. Taylor. "Microbes, microglia, and pain," *Neurobiology of Pain*, 2020 Jan-Jul; 7: 100045 (January 29, 2020). www.ncbi.nlm. nih.gov/pmc/articles/PMC7016021/

[3]   "Can diet heal chronic pain?" Harvard Health Publishing, February 15, 2021, https:// www.health.harvard.edu/pain/can-diet-heal-chronic-pain

[4]   Jo Nijs, et al. "Nutritional intervention in chronic pain: an innovative way of targeting central nervous system sensitization?" *Expert Opinion on Therapeutic Targets*, Vol. 24, 8 (June 28, 2020): 793_803. https://doi.org/10.1080/14728222.2020.1784142

[5]   Jihad Alwarith, et al. "Nutrition Interventions in Rheumatoid Arthritis: The Potential Use of Plant-Based Diets. A Review," *Frontiers in Nutrition*, 6(141), 2019, https://doi. org/10.3389/fnut.2019.00141

[6]   Vincent T. Martin and Vij Brinder. "Diet and Headache: Part 1," *Headache*, 56(9), (2016): 1543–1552. https://doi.org/10.1111/head.12953

[7]   "How to Change Your Diet to Lessen Your Chronic Pain," Health Essentials from Cleveland Clinic, November 9, 2018. https://health.clevelandclinic.org/how-to-change-your-diet-to-lessen-your-chronic-pain/

[8]   Linda Hagfors, et al. "Fat intake and composition of fatty acids in serum phospholipids in a randomized, controlled, Mediterranean dietary intervention study on patients with rheumatoid arthritis," *Nutrition & Metabolism*, 2(26) (2005). https://doi. org/10.1186/1743-7075-2-26

[9]   Yangzie Xie, et al. "Effects of Diet Based on IgG Elimination Combined with Probiotics on Migraine Plus Irritable Bowel Syndrome," *Pain Research & Management*, Vol. 2019, 7890461 (2019), https://doi.org/10.1155/2019/7890461

[10] Martin, op. cit.

[11] Akiko Okifuji, Bradford D. Hare. "The association between chronic pain and obesity," *Journal of Pain Research*, 8, (2015): 399–408. https://doi.org/10.2147/JPR. S55598

[12] James S. Khan, Jennifer M. Hah, Sean C. Mackey. "Effects of smoking on patients with chronic pain: a propensity-weighted analysis on the Collaborative Health Outcomes Information Registry." *Pain*, 160(10), (2019): 2374–2379, https://doi.org/10.1097/j. pain.0000000000001631

[13] Pacharee Manoy, et al. "Vitamin D Supplementation Improves Quality of Life and Physical Performance in Osteoarthritis Patients," *Nutrients*, 2017 Aug; 9(8) (July 26, 2017): 799. www.ncbi.nlm.nih.gov/pmc/articles/PMC5579593/

[14] Ngozi Awa Imaga. "Phytomedicines and nutraceuticals: alternative therapeutics for sickle cell anemia," *The Scientific World Journal*, 2013, 269659 (Feb 2014), https://doi. org/10.1155/2013/269659

[15] Paramita Basu and Arpita Basu. "In Vitro and In Vivo Effects of Flavonoids on Peripheral Neuropathic Pain," *Molecules* (Basel, Switzerland), 25(5), (March 2020): 1171. https:// doi.org/10.3390/molecules25051171

[16] R. Bonakdar. "Complimentary and integrative medicine approaches in chronic pain," [Lecture], Pain Care for Primary Care (PCPC) 2018, San Diego, CA. (November 16–17, 2018).

[17] Sven Haufe, et al. "Low-dose, non-supervised, health insurance-initiated exercise for the treatment and prevention of chronic low back pain in employees. Results from a randomized controlled trial." *PloS One*, 12(6), e0178585,(2017). https://doi. org/10.1371/journal.pone.0178585

[18] Kristin R. Ambrose and Yvonne M. Golightly. "Physical exercise as non-pharmacological treatment of chronic pain: Why and when." *Best Practice & Research: Clinical Rheumatology*, 29(1), (2015): 120–130. https://doi.org/10.1016/j.berh.2015.04.022

Chapter 4

[1] Bryant A. Meyers. *PEMF – The Fifth Element of Health: Learn Why Pulsed Electromagnetic Field (PEMF) Therapy Supercharges Your Health Like Nothing Else!* (Balboa Press, 2013), p 181.

[2] Ibid.

[3] Tommaso Iannitti, et al. "Pulsed electromagnetic field therapy for management of osteoarthritis-related pain, stiffness and physical function: clinical experience in the elderly." *Clinical Interventions in Aging*, 1289, (2013). https://doi.org/10.2147/cia.s35926

[4] W. A. Jorgensen, B. M. Frome, and C. Wallach. "Electrochemical therapy of pelvic pain: effects of pulsed electromagnetic fields (PEMF) on tissue trauma," *European Journal Surgical Supply*, (574) (1994): 83-6. https://pubmed.ncbi.nlm.nih.gov/7531030/

[5] E. Rowe, et al. "A Prospective, randomized, placebo controlled, double-blind study of pelvic electromagnetic therapy for the treatment of chronic pelvic pain syndrome with 1 year of followup," *The Journal of Urology*, Vol. 173, 6 (June 1, 2005): 2044-2047, https://doi.org/10.1097/01.ju.0000158445.68149.38

[6] Boshra Hatef, et al. "The efficiency of pulsed electromagnetic field in refractory migraine headaches: a randomized, single-blinded, placebo-controlled, parallel group," *International Journal of Clinical Trials*, 3(1), (2016):24-31. http://dx.doi.org/10.18203/2349-3259.ijct20160475

[7] Alex W. Thomas, et al. "A randomized, double-blind, placebo-controlled clinical trial using a low-frequency magnetic field in the treatment of musculoskeletal chronic pain." *Pain Research & Management*, 12(4), (2007): 249–258. https://doi.org/10.1155/2007/626072

[8] V. Graak, et al. "Evaluation of the efficacy of pulsed electromagnetic field in the management of patients with diabetic polyneuropathy," *International journal of diabetes in developing countries*, 29(2), (2009): 56–61. https://doi.org/10.4103/0973-3930.53121

[9] Renato Andrade, et al. "Pulsed electromagnetic field therapy effectiveness in low back pain: A systematic review of randomized controlled trials," *Porto Biomedical Journal*, 1(5), (2016): 156–163. https://doi.org/10.1016/j.pbj.2016.09.001

[10] Ziyang Wu, et al. "Efficacy and safety of the pulsed electromagnetic field in osteoarthritis: a meta-analysis." *BMJ Open*, 8(12), e022879, (2018). https://doi.org/10.1136/bmjopen-2018-022879

[11] Gian Luca Bagnato, et al. "Pulsed electromagnetic fields in knee osteoarthritis: a double blind, placebo-controlled, randomized clinical trial," *Rheumatology* (Oxford, England), 55(4), (2016): 755–762. https://doi.org/10.1093/rheumatology/kev426

[12] Erkam Hattapoglu, et al. "Efficiency of pulsed electromagnetic fields on pain, disability, anxiety, depression, and quality of life in patients with cervical disc herniation: a randomized controlled study," *Turkish Journal of Medical Sciences*, 49(4), (2019): 1095–1101. https://doi.org/10.3906/sag-1901-65

13   Gabriel Tan, et al. "Efficacy of selected complementary and alternative medicine interventions for chronic pain," *Journal of Rehabilitation Research and Development*, 44(2), (2007): 195–222. https://doi.org/10.1682/jrrd.2006.06.0063

14   Anthony J. Lisi, et al. "A Pulsed Electromagnetic Field Therapy Device for Non-Specific Low Back Pain: A Pilot Randomized Controlled Trial," *Pain and Therapy*, 8(1), (2019): 133–140. https://doi.org/10.1007/s40122-019-0119-z

15   Thomas, op. cit.

16   Richard H.W. Funk. "Coupling of pulsed electromagnetic fields (PEMF) therapy to molecular grounds of the cell," *American Journal of Translational Research*, 10(5), (2018): 1260–1272. https://pubmed.ncbi.nlm.nih.gov/29887943/

17   Gladys Lai-Ying Cheing, et al. "Pulsed electromagnetic fields (PEMF) promote early wound healing and myofibroblast proliferation in diabetic rats," *BioElectroMagnetics*, 35(3), (2014): 161–169. https://doi.org/10.1002/bem.21832

18   Michael I. Weintraub, et al. "Pulsed electromagnetic fields to reduce diabetic neuropathic pain and stimulate neuronal repair: a randomized controlled trial," *Archives of Physical Medicine and Rehabilitation*, 90(7), (2009): 1102–1109. https://doi.org/10.1016/j.apmr.2009.01.019

19   Patrick Ziegler, et al. "Pulsed Electromagnetic Field Therapy Improves Osseous Consolidation after High Tibial Osteotomy in Elderly Patients-A Randomized, Placebo-Controlled, Double-Blind Trial," *Journal of Clinical Medicine*, 8(11), 2008, (2019). https://doi.org/10.3390/jcm8112008

20   "Difference between PEMFs (Pulsed Electromagnetic Fields) vs TENS (Transcutaneous Electrical Nerve Stimulation)," FlexPulse, June 13, 2020. https://flexpulse.com/

Chapter 5

1   V. P. Wilson. *Janet G. Travell, MD A Daughter's Recollection, Texas Heart Institute Journal* 2003; 30(1) (2003): 8–12. https://www.ncbi.nlm.nih.gov/

2   Trigger Queen. (n.d.) *Segen's Medical Dictionary* (2011). Retrieved July 25, 2020, https://medical-dictionary.thefreedictionary.com/Trigger+Queen

3   Bryan L. Frank. "Neural Therapy," *Physical Medicine and Rehabilitation Clinics of North America*, 10(3), (1999): 573–582. https://doi.org/10.1016/s1047-9651(18)30181-5

4   P. Barbagli,, R. Bollettin, F. Ceccherelli. "Acupuncture (dry needle) versus neural therapy (local anesthesia) in the treatment of benign back pain. Immediate and long-term results," *Minerva Medica*, 94(4 Suppl 1), (2003): 17–25. https://pubmed.ncbi.nlm.nih.gov/15108608/

5   Heidemarie Haller, et al. "Emotional release and physical symptom improvement: a qualitative analysis of self-reported outcomes and mechanisms in patients treated with neural therapy," *BMC Complementary and Alternative Medicine*, 18(1), (2018): 311. https://doi.org/10.1186/s12906-018-2369-4

6   Spernol, R. & Riss, Paul. (1982). Urodynamische Überprüfung der Neuraltherapie bei motorischer und sensorischer Reizblase. *Geburtshilfe Frauenheilkunde*, 42(7). 527-529. 10.1055/s-2008-1036911.

7   Simon Egli, et al. "Long-term results of therapeutic local anesthesia (neural therapy) in 280 referred refractory chronic pain patients," *BMC Complementary and Alternative Medicine*, 15, (2015): 200. https://doi.org/10.1186/s12906-015-0735-z

[8] Gerald R. Harris. "Neural Therapy and Its Role in the Effective Treatment of Chronic Pain," *Practical Pain Management*. (2011). https://www.practicalpainmanagement.com/treatments/complementary/prolotherapy/neural-therapy-its-role-effective-treatment-chronic-pain.

[9] Robert F. Kidd. *Neural Therapy: Applied Neurophysiology and Other Topics* (Robert F. Kidd, 2020).

[10] "Update of 'Neural Therapy: An Overlooked Game Changer for Patients Suffering Chronic Pain?'" *The Free Library*, (2014). Retrieved Aug 6, 2020. from https://www.thefreelibrary.com/Update+of+%22Neural+Therapy%3a+An+Overlooked+Game+Changer+for+Patients...-a0512184950

Chapter 6

[1] Lamberto Re, Gregorio M. Sanchez, Nabil Mawsouf. "Clinical evidence of ozone interaction with pain mediators," *Saudi Medical Journal*, 31(12), (2010): 1363–1367. https://pubmed.ncbi.nlm.nih.gov/21136002/

[2] V. Bocci. *Oxygen-ozone Therapy: A Critical Evaluation* (Springer 2002).

[3] Masaru Sagai and Velio Bocci. "Mechanisms of Action Involved in Ozone Therapy: Is healing induced via a mild oxidative stress?" *Medical Gas Research*, 1(29) (2011). https://doi.org/10.1186/2045-9912-1-29

[4] Carlo Fuccio, et al. "A single subcutaneous injection of ozone prevents allodynia and decreases the over-expression of pro-inflammatory caspases in the orbito-frontal cortex of neuropathic mice," *European Journal of Pharmacology*, 603(1–3), (2009): 42–49. https://doi.org/10.1016/j.ejphar.2008.11.060

[5] Charles Marchand, *The Therapeutical Applications of Hydrozone and Glycozone*, (Wentworth Press, 2016).

[6] V. Bocci, *OZONE A New Medical Drug* (Softcover reprint of hardcover 1st ed. 2005 ed.), (Springer 2010).

[7] *Medical ozone therapy as a potential treatment modality for regeneration of damaged articular cartilage in osteoarthritis.* (2018, May 1). ScienceDirect. https://www.sciencedirect.com/science/article/pii/S1319562X16000498

[8] *Ozone, a Medical Breakthrough?* is available at the time of this writing to watch online for free at https://youtu.be/H3Q7t3XN7X8)

[9] Xu Feng and Li Beiping. "Therapeutic Efficacy of Ozone Injection into the Knee for the Osteoarthritis Patient along with Oral Celecoxib and Glucosamine," *Journal of Clinical and Diagnostic Research: JCDR*, 11(9), (2017): UC01–UC03. https://doi.org/10.7860/JCDR/2017/26065.10533

[10] Torri, G., Della Grazia, A., & Casadei, C. "Clinical Experience in the Treatment of Lumbar Disk Disease, with a Cycle of Lumbar Muscles Injections of an Oxygen + Ozone Mixture." Accessed August 7, 2020. www.biaccabi.com/edocs/um_torri.html

[11] F. Magalhaes, et al. "Ozone therapy as a treatment for low back pain secondary to herniated disc: a systematic review and meta-analysis of randomized controlled trials," (2012). Available from: https://www.ncbi.nlm.nih.gov/books/NBK97675/

[12] Seung Yeop Lee, et al. "Lumbar Stenosis: A Recent Update by Review of Literature," *Asian Spine Journal*, 9(5), (2015): 818–828. https://doi.org/10.4184/asj.2015.9.5.818

[13] J. Baeza-Noci. "Spinal ozone therapy in lumbar spinal stenosis," *International Journal of Ozone Therapy*. 6, (2007): 17-24.

14 Velio Bocci, et al. "The usefulness of ozone treatment in spinal pain," *Drug Design, Development and Therapy*, 9, (2015): 2677–2685. https://doi.org/10.2147/DDDT. S74518

15 Omar Seyam, et al. "Clinical utility of ozone therapy for musculoskeletal disorders," *Medical Gas Research*, 8(3) (2018): 103–110. https://doi.org/10.4103/2045-9912.241075

16 Giulio Peretti. "Shoulder adhesive capsulitis, treatment with oxygen ozone: Technique and results," *Ozone Therapy*, Vol. 2 (2017). https://doi.org/10.4081/ozone.2017.7245

17 M. Doğan, et al. "Effects of high-frequency bio-oxidative ozone therapy in temporomandibular disorder-related pain," *Medical principles and practice: international journal of the Kuwait University, Health Science Centre*, 23(6), (2014:. 507–510. https://doi.org/10.1159/000365355

18 Seyed Ahmad Raeissadat, et al. "An investigation into the efficacy of intra-articular ozone (O2–O3) injection in patients with knee osteoarthritis: a systematic review and meta-analysis," *Journal of Pain Research*, 2018; 11(2018): 2537–2550. https://www.ncbi.nlm.nih.gov/pmc/articles/PMC6207244/

19 Schwartz, A. (2016). Solución Salina Ozonizada (Sso3): Fundamentos Científicos. Revista Española de Ozonoterapia. Vol. 6, No. 1, pp 121-129.

20 Schwartz, A. (2020). *ISCO3 Madrid Declaration on Ozone Therapy (3rd Edition) Digital: English & Spanish*. Https://Isco3.Org/. https://isco3.org/madrid-declaration-on-ozone-therapy-3rd-edition-isco3/

Chapter 7

1 Erminia Mariani and Lia Pulsatelli. "Platelet Concentrates in Musculoskeletal Medicine," *International journal of molecular sciences*, 21(4), (2020): 1328. https://doi.org/10.3390/ijms21041328

2 Paul J. Christo. *Aches and Gains: A Comprehensive Guide to Overcoming Your Pain (1st ed.)*, (Bull Publishing Company, 2017), 279.

3 Nathan Wei. *The Book on PRP: An easy to understand "Consumer's Guide" to Understanding How Platelet-rich Plasma Is Used to Treat Problems Such As Tendonitis, Ligament Damage, Bursitis, Fasciitis, and Other Related Disorders* (CreateSpace Independent Publishing Platform, 2010).

4 Ibid.

Chapter 8

1 World Health Organization: WHO. (2016, April 8). *Headache disorders*. World Health Organization. https://www.who.int/news-room/fact-sheets/detail/headache-disorders

2 GBD 2016 Headache Collaborators. "Global, regional, and national burden of migraine and tension-type headache, 1990–2016: a systematic analysis for the Global Burden of Disease Study 2016," *The Lancet* (November 2018). https://doi.org/10.1016/S1474-4422(18)30322-3

3 Simona Sacco, et al. "Migraine in women: the role of hormones and their impact on vascular diseases," *The Journal of Headache and Pain*, 13(3), (2012): 177–189. https://doi.org/10.1007/s10194-012-0424-y

4   Anna E. Kirkland, Gabrielle L. Sarlo, Kathleen F. Holton. "The Role of Magnesium
     in Neurological Disorders," *MDPI* (June 6, 2018). https://www.mdpi.com/2072-
     6643/10/6/730/htm
5   E. Estemalik and S. Tepper. "Preventive treatment in migraine and the new US
     guidelines," *Neuropsychiatric Disease and Treatment*, 9, (2013): 709–720. https://doi.
     org/10.2147/NDT.S33769
6   Mustafa Calik, et al. "The association between serum vitamin B_{12} deficiency and tension-
     type headache in Turkish children," *Neurological Sciences: Official Journal of the Italian
     Neurological Society and of the Italian Society of Clinical Neurophysiology*, 39(6) (2018):
     1009–1014. https://doi.org/10.1007/s10072-018-3286-5
7   Claire E. Lunde and Christine B. Sieberg. "Walking the Tightrope: A Proposed Model
     of Chronic Pain and Stress," *Frontiers in Neuroscience*, 14(270) (2020). https://doi.
     org/10.3389/fnins.2020.00270

Chapter 9

1   "Chronic Back Pain," Health Policy Institute. (February 13, 2019). https://hpi.
     georgetown.edu/backpain/
2   Ahmed Mohamed Elshiwi, et al. "Effect of pulsed electromagnetic field on nonspecific
     low back pain patients: a randomized controlled trial," *Brazilian Journal of Physical
     Therapy*, 23(3), (2019): 244–249. https://doi.org/10.1016/j.bjpt.2018.08.004
3   N. S. Atalay, et al. "Comparison of efficacy of neural therapy and physical therapy in
     chronic low back pain," *African Journal of Traditional, Complementary, and Alternative
     Medicines: AJTCAM*, 10(3), (2013): 431–435. https://doi.org/10.4314/ajtcam.v10i3.8
4   Alessio Biazzo, Andrea S. Corriero, and Norberto Confalonieri. "Intramuscular oxygen-
     ozone therapy in the treatment of low back pain," *Acta Biomedica*, 89(1) (2018): 41–46.
     https://doi.org/10.23750/abm.v89i1.5315
5   H. Nazlıkul, et al. "Evaluation of neural therapy effect in patients with piriformis
     syndrome," *Journal of Back and Musculoskeletal Rehabilitation*, 31(6), (2018): 1105–
     1110. https://doi.org/10.3233/bmr-170980
6   Massimo Gallucci, et al. "Sciatica: Treatment with Intradiscal and Intraforaminal
     Injections of Steroid and Oxygen-Ozone versus Steroid Only," *Radiology*, 242(3) (2007):
     907–913. https://doi.org/10.1148/radiol.2423051934
7   Suja Mohammed and James Yu. "Platelet-rich plasma injections: an emerging therapy for
     chronic discogenic low back pain," *Journal of Spine Surgery* (Hong Kong), 4(1) (2018):
     115–122. https://doi.org/10.21037/jss.2018.03.04
8   Xiaodong Pang, Hong Yang, and Baogan Peng. "Human umbilical cord mesenchymal
     stem cell transplantation for the treatment of chronic discogenic low back pain," *Pain
     Physician*, 17(4) (2014): E525–E530. https://pubmed.ncbi.nlm.nih.gov/25054402/

Chapter 10

1   Steven P. Cohen and W. Michael Hooten. "Advances in the diagnosis and management
     of neck pain," *BMJ*, (August 14, 2017). https://www.bmj.com/content/358/bmj.j3221
2   Merve Karakaş and Haydar Gök. "Effectiveness of pulsed electromagnetic field therapy
     on pain, functional status, and quality of life in patients with chronic non-specific neck

pain: A prospective, randomized-controlled study," *Turkish Journal of Physical Medicine and Rehabilitation*, 66(2) (2020): 140–146. https://doi.org/10.5606/tftrd.2020.5169

3   Angela Cadogan, et al. "A prospective study of shoulder pain in primary care: prevalence of imaged pathology and response to guided diagnostic blocks," *BMC Musculoskeletal Disorders*, 12, (2011): 119. https://doi.org/10.1186/1471-2474-12-119

4   Diego Galace de Freitas, et al. "Pulsed Electromagnetic Field and Exercises in Patients with Shoulder Impingement Syndrome: A Randomized, Double-Blind, Placebo-Controlled Clinical Trial," *Archives of Physical Medicine and Rehabilitation*, 95(2), (2014): 45–352. https://doi.org/10.1016/j.apmr.2013.09.022

5   Seyam, op. cit.

6   Dong-wook Rha, et al. "Comparison of the therapeutic effects of ultrasound-guided platelet-rich plasma injection and dry needling in rotator cuff disease: a randomized controlled trial," *Clinical Rehabilitation*, 27(2), (2013): 113–122. https://doi.org/10.1177/0269215512448388

7   Dimitrios Giotis, et al. "Effectiveness of Biologic Factors in Shoulder Disorders," *The Open Orthopaedics Journal*, 11, (2017): 163–182. https://doi.org/10.2174/1874325001711010163

8   Uyen-sa D. T. Nguyen, et al. "Increasing prevalence of knee pain and symptomatic knee osteoarthritis: survey and cohort data," *Annals of internal medicine*, *155*(11), (2011): 725–732. https://doi.org/10.7326/0003-4819-155-11-201112060-00004

9   Bagnato, op cit.

10 Feng, op cit.

11 Krishnan Chakravarthy, et al. "Stem Cell Therapy for Chronic Pain Management: Review of Uses, Advances, and Adverse Effects," *Pain Physician*, 20(4) (2017): 293–305. https://pubmed.ncbi.nlm.nih.gov/28535552/

12 Jose Matas, et al. "Umbilical Cord-Derived Mesenchymal Stromal Cells (MSCs) for Knee Osteoarthritis: Repeated MSC Dosing Is Superior to a Single MSC Dose and to Hyaluronic Acid in a Controlled Randomized Phase I/II Trial," *Stem Cells Translational Medicine*, 8(3) (2019): 215–224. https://doi.org/10.1002/sctm.18-0053

Chapter 11

1   *Fibromyalgia*. (n.d.). Centers for Disease Control and Prevention. www.cdc.gov/arthritis/basics/fibromyalgia.htm

2   Kevin C. Fleming. "Is fibromyalgia hereditary?" Mayo Clinic (September 6, 2017). https://www.mayoclinic.org/diseases-conditions/fibromyalgia/expert-answers/is-fibromyalgia-hereditary/faq20058091#:%7E:text=Fibromyalgia%20isn't%20passed%20directly,which%20no%20one%20has%20fibromyalgia.

3   Naomi M. Shupak, et al. "Exposure to a Specific Pulsed Low-Frequency Magnetic Field: A Double-Blind Placebo-Controlled Study of Effects on Pain Ratings in Rheumatoid Arthritis and Fibromyalgia Patients," *Pain Research and Management*, 11(2) (2006): 85–90. https://doi.org/10.1155/2006/842162

4   Brenda P. Longas Vélez. "Ozone therapy, a supplement for patients with fibromyalgia," *Revista Española de Ozonoterapia*. Vol. 4, No. 1 (2014): 39-49.

5   Luminita Labusca, Florin Zugun-Eloae, and Kaveh Mashayekhi. "Stem cells for the treatment of musculoskeletal pain," *World Journal of Stem Cells*, 7(1) (2015): 96–105. https://doi.org/10.4252/wjsc.v7.i1.96

6   Esra Semiz, et al. "Serum cortisol and dehydroepiandrosterone-sulfate levels after balneotherapy and physical therapy in patients with fibromyalgia," *Saudi Medical Journal*, 37(5) (2016): 544–550. https://doi.org/10.15537/smj.2016.5.15032

7   Jarred Younger, et al. "Low-dose naltrexone for the treatment of fibromyalgia: findings of a small, randomized, double-blind, placebo-controlled, counterbalanced, crossover trial assessing daily pain levels," *Arthritis and rheumatism*, 65(2) (2013): 529–538. https://doi.org/10.1002/art.37734

8   Amanda M. Brandow, Rebecca A. Farley, and Julie A. Panepinto. "Neuropathic pain in patients with sickle cell disease," *Pediatric Blood & Cancer*, 61(3), (2014): 512–517. https://doi.org/10.1002/pbc.24838

9   *About Sickle Cell Disease*. (n.d.). NIH National Human Genome Research Institute. https://www.genome.gov/Genetic-Disorders/Sickle-Cell-Disease

10 *Who Gets MS?* (n.d.). National Multiple Sclerosis Society. https://www.nationalmssociety.org/What-is-MS/Who-Gets-MS

11 Brandi Koskie. "Multiple Sclerosis: Facts, Statistics, and You," Healthline. (March 9, 2020). https://www.healthline.com/health/multiple-sclerosis/facts-statistics-infographic#1

12 A. Hochsprung, et al. "Effectiveness of monopolar dielectric transmission of pulsed electromagnetic fields for multiple sclerosisâ related pain: a pilot study," *Neuroliga*, Vol. 36, No. 6, 433–439. https://doi.org/10.1016/j.nrleng.2018.03.003

13 Robin Gordon Gibson and Sheila L. M. Gibson. "Neural Therapy in the Treatment of Multiple Sclerosis," *The Journal of Alternative and Complementary Medicine*, 5(6), (1999): 543–552. https://doi.org/10.1089/acm.1999.5.543

14 F. Molinari, et al. "Ozone autohemotherapy induces long-term cerebral metabolic changes in multiple sclerosis patients," *International Journal of Immunopathology and Pharmacology*, 27(3) (2014): 379–389. https://doi.org/10.1177/039463201402700308

15 Javed Ameli, et al. "Mechanisms of pathophysiology of blood vessels in patients with multiple sclerosis treated with ozone therapy: a systematic review," *Acta Biomedica: Atenei Parmensis*, 90(3) (2019): 213–217. https://doi.org/10.23750/abm.v90i3.7265

16 Beth Longware Duff. "Shingles and PHN by the Numbers," *Drug Topics* (November 1, 2018). https://www.drugtopics.com/view/shingles-and-phn-numbers

17 Ibid.

18 Fred Hui, et al. "A randomized controlled trial of a multifaceted integrated complementary-alternative therapy for chronic herpes zoster-related pain," *Alternative Medicine Review: A Journal of Clinical Therapeutic*, 17(1) (2012): 57–68. https://pubmed.ncbi.nlm.nih.gov/22502623/

19 Bin Hu, et al. "The effect and safety of ozone autohemotherapy combined with pharmacological therapy in postherpetic neuralgia," *Journal of Pain Research*, 11 (2018): 1637–1643. https://doi.org/10.2147/JPR.S154154

20 *National Diabetes Statistics Report, 2020*. Centers for Disease Control and Prevention. Retrieved September 4, 2020, from https://www.cdc.gov/diabetes/data/statistics-report/index.html

21 Kelsey Juster-Switlyk and A. Gordon Smith. "Updates in diabetic peripheral neuropathy," *F1000Research*, 5, F1000 Faculty Rev-738 (2016). https://doi.org/10.12688/f1000research.7898.1

22 Evangelos Agathos, et al. "Effect of α-lipoic acid on symptoms and quality of life in patients with painful diabetic neuropathy," *The Journal of International Medical Research*, 46(5), (2018): 1779–1790. https://doi.org/10.1177/0300060518756540

23 C. Norman Shealy and Sergey Sorin. "Pulsed Electromagnetic Field Therapy: Innovative Treatment for Diabetic Neuropathy," *Practical Pain Management* (2016). https://www.practicalpainmanagement.com/treatments/interventional/stimulators/pulsed-electromagnetic-field-therapy-innovative-treatment

Chapter 12

1   Alexander M. Dydyk and Nishant. "Chronic Pelvic Pain," StatPearls (Updated June 23, 2020). https://www.ncbi.nlm.nih.gov/books/NBK554585/

2   Manish K. Singh. "Chronic Pelvic Pain in Women: Background, Pathophysiology, Epidemiology," Medscape (November 9, 2019). https://emedicine.medscape.com/article/258334-overview#:%7E:text=Chronic%20pelvic%20pain%20is%20a,10%25%20are%20for%20pelvic%20pain

3   Iris Kerin Orbuch and Amy Stein. *Beating Endo: How to Reclaim Your Life from Endometriosis* (Illustrated ed.) (Harper Wave, June 21, 2019).

4   Tyler L. Overholt, et al. "Pulsed Electromagnetic Field Therapy as a Complementary Alternative for Chronic Pelvic Pain Management in an Interstitial Cystitis/Bladder Pain Syndrome Patient [Slides]," *Case Reports in Urology* (December 26, 2019). https://pubmed.ncbi.nlm.nih.gov/31949970/

5   J. Curtis Nickel. "Injection therapy for urologic chronic pelvic pain: Lessons learned," *Canadian Urological Association Journal* (6 Suppl 3), (2018): S186–S188. https://doi.org/10.5489/cuaj.5333

6   R. M. Kronenberg, S. M. Ludin, and L. Fischer. "Severe Case of Chronic Pelvic Pain Syndrome: Recovery after Injection of Procaine into the Vesicoprostatic Plexus-Case Report and Discussion of Pathophysiology and Mechanisms of Action," *Case Reports in Urology*, 2018, 9137215 (2018). https://doi.org/10.1155/2018/9137215

7   Christopher P. Smith. "Male chronic pelvic pain: An update," *IJU: Journal of the Urological Society of India*, 32(1), (2016): 34–39. https://doi.org/10.4103/0970-1591.173105

8   Ibid.

Chapter 13

1   Thomas G. Weiser, et al. "An estimation of the global volume of surgery: a modelling strategy based on available data," *The Lancet*, 372(9633), (2008): 139–144. https://doi.org/10.1016/s0140-6736(08)60878-8

2   Darin Correll. "Chronic postoperative pain: recent findings in understanding and management," *F1000Research*, 6, (2017): 1054. https://doi.org/10.12688/f1000research.11101.1

3   Ibid.

4   Tom Seymour. "Direct vs. indirect inguinal hernias," *MedicalNewsToday*. (May 17, 2017). https://www.medicalnewstoday.com/articles/317489#What-is-an-inguinal-hernia

5   W. A. Macrae. "Chronic post-surgical pain: 10 years on," *British Journal of Anaesthesia*, 101(1) (2008): 77–86. https://doi.org/10.1093/bja/aen099

6   L. Macdonald, et al. "Long-term follow-up of breast cancer survivors with post-mastectomy pain syndrome," *British Journal of Cancer*, 92(2), (2005): 225–230. https://doi.org/10.1038/sj.bjc.6602304

7   Maryam Khooshideh, et al. "Pulsed Electromagnetic Fields for Postsurgical Pain Management in Women Undergoing Cesarean Section: A Randomized, Double-Blind, Placebo-controlled Trial," *The Clinical Journal of Pain*, 33(2), (2017): 142–147. https://doi.org/10.1097/AJP.0000000000000376

8   Shu-Hung Huang, et al. "Platelet-Rich Plasma Injection in Burn Scar Areas Alleviates Neuropathic Scar Pain," *International Journal of Medical Sciences*, 15(3) (2018): 238–247. https://doi.org/10.7150/ijms.22563

About the Author

Karima Hirani, MD, MPH, is a board-certified family physician with a Master of Public Health degree in nutrition. Dr. Hirani earned her master's degree from the UCLA School of Public Health and graduated from USC Medical School, where she taught from 2007 to 2014. Dr. Hirani completed her postgraduate training at Long Beach Memorial Family Medicine Residency Training Program. She also holds board certification in clinical homeopathy, a lifelong dream.

Dr. Hirani stated, "I knew from the time I was seven that I wanted to be a doctor although I didn't exactly know why at the time. I was born in Nairobi, Kenya, where my mother was a member of the American Red Cross. She would take me on all her trips to feed the needy, which were great adventures at my young age. My grandmother was an herbalist back in India, so I guess wanting to help people runs in my DNA."

In 2001, Dr. Hirani founded the Hirani Integrative Medical Center in Culver City, California. The practice focuses on complementary and alternative medicine (CAM) and integrative medicine. "My approach to pain management is a combination of therapies, which I call The Golden Triad for Pain Relief.™ It features three advanced methods that are foundational to our successful treatments at the Hirani Integrative Medical Center—pulsed electromagnetic field (PEMF) therapy, neural trigger point therapy, and oxygen-ozone therapy." Dr. Hirani is expert in these.

The Hirani Integrative Medical Center specializes in treating adults with chronic illnesses, chronic pain, and immune disorders. Dr. Hirani has also had significant success in treating children with autism. Additionally, her clinic offers platelet-rich plasma (PRP) and stem cells for pain relief as well as surgical-free facelifts and cosmetic work.

"As long as there is hope, I am committed to searching for alternative pain solutions. For many patients, we need to take a deeper look into the mechanisms of chronic illness and pain, asking whether there is a nutritional deficiency or autoimmune, hormonal, or environmental component that's triggering a patient's persistent chronic pain. The cutting-edge therapies we use are an example of our dedication to leaving no stone unturned for our patients."

Dr. Hirani is a lead organizer at ICSC Food Pantry in Korea Town in Los Angeles, also feeding the homeless on Skid Row every week. Dr. Hirani also volunteers her time to educate undeserved communities throughout Los Angeles on various health topics such as nutrition, diabetes, and heart disease.

"My patients inspired me to share with others like them that there is hope for pain sufferers. Ideally, this first book is for chronic pain sufferers who have lost all hope as well as those who are the opposite—who refuse to accept that pain is a life sentence. So, if you haven't had any success with traditional pain treatments, or if you've had too many side effects from pain medications and treatments, then this book was written for you."

It will soon be followed by books on building the immune system during COVID and diet for chronic pain. A future collaborative study of male pelvic pain is also in the works.

After treating more than a thousand patients with successful outcomes, Dr. Hirani states this with confidence:

"You don't need to let another day go by with pain—that is our mission!"

Index